Suicide Risk in the Bay Area

Suicide Risk in the Bay Area

A Guide for Families, Physicians, Therapists & Other Professionals

Eli Merritt, M.D.

Published by Compass Health Books
San Francisco, CA

Disclaimer:
The information contained in this book is provided to aid and assist families, physicians, therapists, and other professionals in care navigation, access to care, and suicide prevention in the Bay Area. It does not constitute medical or legal advice. Standards for suicide risk assessment, hospital services, mobile crisis access, and hotline phone numbers change frequently. Users of the book should confirm availability and appropriateness of services independently and in all cases should call 911 without delay in the event of a psychiatric emergency.

Book design and typesetting by Tom Comitta
Printed in the United States

*Dedicated to patients, families, and friends
affected by suicide and suicide risk*

Contents

Acknowledgements

In writing this book I owe a debt of gratitude to many people. To Tom Comitta, artist and book producer who designed the cover and layout and energized the project from from concept to completion with wit, intelligence, and enthusiasm. Without Tom, there would be no book. To David Herschorn, photographer and creative thinker who launched Merritt Mental Health with me in 2014 and encouraged the book from its clumsy beginnings. To Cynthia Shiraev, Dan Benbow, and Caleb Feigin, tireless researchers who investigated and compiled resources. To Caleb Beckwith, copy editor, Taylor Lord, intern, and readers Eve Meyer and Robert Solley who provided valuable insight and caught oversights.

Thoughtful friends took hours of time to *Talk About It* with me. Harrison Hobart and I played tennis on Sundays on the Embarcadero, followed by long conversations about the book, American culture, and existential perspectives on suicide risk. Amy Atkinson, through encouraging words and the gift of books and radiant smiles, imbued *esprit* into this book. Jay O'Connor, master of brainstorming, helped me to conceive of *Suicide Risk in the Bay Area* as the beginning of a movement, not as the end of a research project. Sam Naifeh, over coffees and lunches, taught me about the dark link between addiction and suicide while beaming brightly all the while about the importance of the book. Other friends I would like to thank for their support and input are Mark Atkinson, Heather Corcoran, Blyth Lord, Julie Benello, Michael Johns, Pete Chung, Burns Jones, Chris Donohoe, Robin Donohoe, Peter Fry, Ben Humphreys, Lisa Humphreys, Jack Wieland, Jim Fuller, Marsha Vande Berg, Jordana Tann, Jonathan Tann, Jon Shayne, Sam Hocking, Jennifer Hocking, Kathryn Huarte, Shelly Kasowitz, Janell Hobart, Jeanne Darrah, David Brodwin, Fran Miller, Lawrence Chang, Sean Bourke, Quincy Smith, Kat Kantz, Ricky Seminsky, Leslie McAllister, Andrew McAllister, Tom Clayton, Kathy Meadowcroft, Tom Meadowcroft, Erin Steere, Jim Schmidt, and many others.

Colleagues and experts in the fields of psychiatry, addiction, and forensics rallied to my support. I thank you all: Renee Binder, Alan Schatzberg, Adam Strassberg, David Sheff, Randall Hagar, Anne Fleming, Winston Chung, Mark Berl, Rona Hu, Esme Shaller, Nazneen Bahrassa, Jan Yaffe, Courtney Brown, Renée Binder, Kate Northcott, Randall Hagar, Marv Firestone, Fancher Larson, Bob Cabaj, Andrew Booty, Melissa Nau, Rick Cicinelli, Caroline Fleck, Emily Schermerhorn, Kevin Briggs, David Pines, Cortne Bui, Ryan Ayers, Tracie Ruble, Mark O'Brien, Robin Cooper, Larry Lurie, Mimi Winsberg, Yelena Zalkina, Ira Steinman, Ceci Walken, Karen Palamos, Stephen Hall, Bridget Whitlow, Alice Tanner, Scott Gorman, Katie Barry, Russ Monroe, David Hull, Paul Muller, Ashleigh Servadio, Sharon Epel, Steve Walsh, Chris Capelle, Victor Yalom, Howard Kornfeld, Meghan Freebeck, Courtney Brown, Stephen Marks, Paul Abramson, Jacqueline Perlmutter, Dick Shadoan, Robin Apple, Harvey Dondershine, Jeb Berkeley, Brian Mohlenhoff, Randy Weingarten, Joanne Cohen, Tim Sinclair, David Becker, Robin Stuart, Don Summers, Kyra Minninger, Ken Braslow, Zena Potash, Kira Olson, Roberta Corson, Kathleen Dong, Athena Papadakos, Patti Pike, Cathryn Lewis, Amy Tyson, Elizabeth Stuart, Alan Altman, Brad Engwald, Peter Carpenter, Descartes Li, Andy Erkis, Emery Fu, Shemeta Hankerson, Ralph Fenn, Anisha Patel-Dunn, Roy Curry, and Charles Saldanha. I dedicate this book to the memory of one colleague, Alan Sklar, my kind, wise mentor at Stanford during my training there.

And, of course, my patients. There is no job on the planet, I believe, so meaningful as mine. Thank you for taking risks and trusting me to be a fellow traveler and guide.

My family. Thank you dad, Stroud, Louise, Kendall, Uncle John Jay, other cousins, aunts, and uncles in Tennessee. And my great Spanish family in Oviedo. You all seemed to be a cheering squad, and, in so cheering, you once again taught me just what a family is supposed to be.

No one in my life has supported my writing so much as my wife, Rosana. Her loving patience and can-do spirit are unequaled by any other. Only she fully understands the long road taken by me from the banks of the Mississippi River and the Virginia home of James Madison to the shores of *Suicide Risk in the Bay Area.*

Finally, three children: my niece Fields and my two sons Ale and Cameron. Fields, just thinking about you from afar lights up my day. Keep on being you. And Ale and Cameron. You too taught me how to *Talk About It.* Your mere existence fills me with joy. You three are, by far, the brightest stars in my universe.

Foreword

This unique and concise book brings to mind a story shared by Nora Volkow, M.D., Director of the National Institute on Drug Abuse, at the 2015 annual meeting of the American Psychiatric Association. Dr. Volkow related a memory of being summoned to her mother's deathbed and learning new information about the life and death of her grandfather.

"I need to tell you something I've never spoken to you about," her mother, weak from a long fight with cancer, said. Dr. Volkow had been told as a child that her grandfather had died suddenly from cardiovascular disease. Now, at the end of her life, Dr. Volkow's mother revealed the truth: Her grandfather, who had long suffered from alcoholism, took his own life.

Dr. Volkow's mother had never told her about the cause of death because of shame and stigma. As Dr. Merritt reveals in the pages that follow, he, like Dr. Volkow, has had personal experience with suicide. When he was six years old, his mother committed suicide. He describes the shame experienced by his family. It is from this family experience and his work as a psychiatrist that Dr. Merritt was inspired to write this book.

In this book, Dr. Merritt advocates for an important message that will help decrease stigma. When it comes to suicide, he tells us simply, "Talk About It." He is correct. The most powerful medicines we have to combat the shame and stigma surrounding psychiatric illness, addiction, and suicide are courage, honesty, and open dialogue.

Suicide Risk in the Bay Area deserves to be on the desks of every mental health professional who lives and works in the Bay Area. It is also a valuable resource for student health centers and occupational health centers. It is an innovative work that is, in fact, two-books-in-one. On the one hand, it is a valuable reference guide to hotlines, mobile crisis services, hospitals, treatment centers, and other suicide-related resources. Yet, throughout the same pages, the book provides concise step-by-step educational modules in suicide risk assessment and management.

Suicide Risk in the Bay Area is a new concept in suicide prevention worthy of emulation nationwide. Imagine a book, or mobile app, called *Suicide Risk in New York City*—or Los Angeles, Chicago, Philadelphia, Houston, Nashville, Washington, D.C. Mental health professionals everywhere should promote the *Talk About It* campaign and have readily available resources and referrals for suicide prevention.

Renée Binder, M.D.
President, American Psychiatric Association
Arlington, Virginia
October 2015

Introduction

This book, which grows out of events both professional and personal in my life, first surfaced as a necessity when I decided to launch a mental health consultancy with a mission to help patients and families get connected with the right care. After fifteen years of practice, I came to the conclusion that our mental health system is a fragmented "non-system" of potholes and pitfalls that adds stress to the lives of those seeking care long before it helps them. The non-system has become so complex, so diverse, so expensive, and, in some areas, so inaccessible that, paradoxically, it has become an underlying cause of suffering and anguish.

Over the decades my own experience as a doctor, and occasional patient, taught me this truth about mental health care. Colleagues, family, and friends validated the point. So did my patients, especially the most ill among them. Their voices mattered most of all in my decision to start a care navigation practice. They and their family members need help not only with compromised mental health and addiction but with navigating the labyrinth of diagnoses, doctors, therapists, hospitals, programs, and insurance barriers facing them.

So I decided to launch a consultancy to help them find their way. However, before I could go forward, I had to figure out two critical things.

One was substance abuse and addiction, and the other was suicide risk. I am a well-schooled psychiatrist, but few lay people actually understand how poorly trained most health professionals are in these two essential—needless to say, life-and-death—domains of health and illness. The reason, at least in part, is that we are still emerging from a Middle Age stigma and shame on both fronts.

To maximally help patients and family members as a guide to the non-system, I concluded, I first had to delve deeply into these twin disciplines and improve myself. I started with substance abuse and addiction and moved from there into suicide risk.

Certainly, a desperately-needed, lifesaving book could be written called *Addiction Treatment in the Bay Area: A Guide for Families, Physicians, Therapists, and Other Professionals*. I have thought about writing it. It should be written.

My more immediate and deeper personal calling, however, lay in the area of suicide risk.

Personal Experience

These many professional motivations behind my interest in suicide risk are accurate and true. But not uncommonly there is a story-within-the-story—a personal motivation, that is, or tragedy of some kind, behind a newfound professional devotion. In my case, it was two such galvanizing events separated by a span of thirty years.

The first occurred seven years after I went into practice in San Francisco. A fine, promising young patient of mine, a 26-year-old with bipolar disorder and substance abuse, had lately been doing better. He was in love and told me, for the first time, that he hoped to marry. Soon after, I left town with my family for a long ski weekend in Tahoe. Two days later his girlfriend broke up with him, and he drove to the Golden Gate Bridge and jumped to his death.

My reaction was everything the grief literature foretells—shock, disbelief, numbness, sadness, depression, guilt, and bargaining the death away somehow. Since I am a doctor living in a notoriously litigious society, there was also a large dose of superadded fear about being blamed in a lawsuit.

As the months advanced, I decided that psychiatry was no longer the right field for me. I wanted out. It stung too much. I daydreamed about career change. I had always wanted to attend the Yale Law School—not to be a lawyer, mind you, but simply for the intellectual pleasure of being there—and I almost applied.

In the end, the death of my patient combined psychologically with a significant death from my childhood to shift my course. After several years of soul-searching and hard study, I came to a place of greater peace with those things I cannot control, suicide among them. I decided that I must do better in the clinical assessment and management of suicide risk, but, as critically, I realized that I can only do my best.

I can only do my best. This insight swept me with a settled, freeing feeling. It gave me confidence and, more vitally, humility. It helped release me from the trappings of fear, shame, and guilt that so often beset families touched by suicide.

That's the second part of the story-within-the-story. The childhood death I mentioned was of my mother to suicide. I was six years old. My sister was seven. My brother was eight. She was bipolar. There was a readily accessible firearm in the house. It seems ineffable and sad, and it was.

Yet the thing that hit us children the hardest, until identity crises struck in young adulthood, was not sadness. It was shame. The shame was bright red, everywhere, and penetrating. Imagine. It was the 1970s, and it was suicide in the southern city of Franklin, Tennessee. My father was a prominent lawyer. My grandparents on both sides were members of the club and, shall we say, socially conscious. It was, of course, also the era before the biological model of mental illness had enlightened us about the outsized role genetics play in depression, bipolar disorder, and suicide.

My other most vivid memory of that time as a young child is one of waiting and waiting—waiting in the kitchen for her to come home through the large wood-paneled side door. No one had ever permanently disappeared in my life, only temporarily. Samuel Beckett's *Waiting for Godot* later took on special meaning for me.

In the play, the long-awaited Godot never comes. Neither did my mother.

So, as you can see, there was a double effect of my patient's suicide. It reawakened old feelings and complexes related to none other than the mother figure of Freudian lore. I have lectured about an entity called the "suicide complex"—not the one inside the person who might commit suicide, but the one inside the treating professional or family member. It's that bundle of denial, anxiety, guilt, fear, dread, and helplessness that inadvertently redirects a doctor or therapist away from talking adequately about suicide with someone who, in fact, desperately needs to talk about it.

Suffice it to say, I learned about the concept of suicide complex by studying my own.

As it turns out, Freud was right about loss. It cuts to the bone. It wrenches the heart. Suicide, with its stigma and enigma, makes death all the more twisting and hidden. Those who have lost a family member, friend, or patient to suicide understand this added layer of complexity: the shrinking feelings of shame and blame that accompany this special form of death.

Friends & Family

The call came in shortly after 2 pm on a Wednesday. I was in Nashville visiting family during the summertime, driving into town from the outskirts. The father who left the voicemail said he wished to speak to me as soon as possible about his 16 year-old daughter who had recently been hospitalized at John Muir Hospital in Concord.

Heeding the call, I pulled over to the side of the road and parked, facing head-on the bizarre green-and-white mermaid logo of Starbucks at a nearby strip mall. I dialed the father back, and he answered. He was from Palo Alto. He had gotten my name from a friend who was the patient of a Stanford doctor who knew me well from residency days.

Wisely, the father was conducting due diligence about the best next step for his daughter upon discharge from the hospital. In the outpatient world, she already had a therapist, a psychiatrist, and an eating disorder specialist. Added to this, she was enrolled twice weekly in a Dialectical Behavior Therapy group.

Should she return to this therapeutic framework, he asked, or enter a residential treatment program or a "PHP or IOP"?

PHP stands for partial hospital program, IOP for intensive outpatient program. Both are day programs that offer a combination

---

Talking about suicide is challenging, to say the least. It's not a panacea. However, it is a vital mission of suicide prevention and a vital mission of this book.

---

of therapy, education, and structure—all extremely helpful in healing from an acute emotional crisis or chronic illness. PHPs run about 20 hours per week, IOPs about half that.

The daughter, whom I shall call Nancy, had been under psychological care in one form or another since age 10. She had been diagnosed with depression and anxiety and took a low dose of Zoloft daily. A junior in high school, she made excellent grades. Nonetheless, her father said, she worried constantly about tests, college applications, and friends.

Three days before our call, Nancy told her mother that she could not stop thinking about suicide. It had been going on for days. She had visions of cutting her wrists with a box cutter her father kept in the garage for breaking down cardboard for recycling.

After this, he told me something more concerning.

"I've made my peace with death," Nancy apparently said in a depressed manner, her head low, eyes averted.

An hour later the mother and father took her to the emergency department for evaluation. She was admitted, and that same morning of our phone call a social worker told the parents that she would probably be released within 48 hours.

"Have you talked to her about it and told her how you feel?" I asked the father.

"Talked to her about what?" he responded.

"Her death by suicide and how it would affect you."

He was taken aback, even a bit put off, by the nature of my question.

"No, I haven't," he answered.

During that phone call and one more the following day, I helped the father to understand the intricacies of psychiatric care, and I honestly shared what my personal decision-making process would look like if it were one of my two sons who was hospitalized under similar circumstances. I educated him about the genetics of depression and grounded him in the science of "gene-environment interactionism," the most accurate model for understanding depressive illnesses and suicide risk.

But what mattered most in our conversations was my specific recommendation that he have an open-hearted, loving conversation about suicide with his daughter.

I counseled him to Talk About It. My suggestion was that he take out time for contemplation and get in touch how he would feel if she were gone. He should find a quiet place and go there with a few simple tools, pen and paper. On them he should write down his thoughts and feelings. He would feel pangs of grief, probably, and that was okay. In one sense, that was the point.

Then, after free writing, he should prune the page of everything extraneous, distilling his flow of sentiments down to a single loving essence.

Later, whenever he felt ready, at a time when his daughter was nearby, at a time when he felt soft and tender, even tearful, he should go to her and talk about it.

I recommended that he share his essence and then listen. Talking about it is really about good listening—listening with warmth, love and understanding, no matter what is said, no matter the intensity of the urge in the listener to correct, teach, or lecture.

Listen. Empathize. Validate. These constitute a matchless triad. Then listen some more. Empathize some more. Validate some more. Don't be strong. Don't instruct. Don't fix anything, especially feelings.

In fact, don't talk much (only a little). Instead, be vulnerable. Show your fear and pain. Show your love and sadness. Tears, the stuff of love, help form connection and, I believe, save lives.

Finally, when you have listened long and well, end the listening with a hug and repeat your essence one last time.

Good listening, empathy, love, and connection stand together as a powerful gateway to suicide prevention. It's not the only pathway we have to save lives, certainly. We have great medications, therapies, and other treatments. But it is infinitely the most important—and the most overlooked. Talking about it in this special way, that is, speaking from the softest, most vulnerable places of the heart, often ignites profound emotional shifts in someone who is lost in a dark woods. Talking about it in this way, once and again, restores lost hope.

At the end of the two phone calls, Nancy's father was grateful. Several weeks later we were in touch again, and he let me know that he and his wife had spoken to his daughter about suicide risk. They sat down with Nancy in her bedroom after the writing exercise. The essence they developed, he said, was a commitment do *anything for the sake of her health*. She could get C's and D's. It didn't matter. She could change schools. She could take a gap year before college. The father told her he would take a leave of absence from his job to be with her. The parents would get their own therapeutic help. The whole family, perhaps, could take a hiatus from the Bay Area and go on a self-fashioned one-year sabbatical.

Stated in another way, the essence Nancy's parents communicated was that nothing in the world was more important to them than Nancy just as she is and that nothing in the world would cause them more lifelong hurt and sadness than her death by suicide.

They would move mountains to keep her alive. They did not just entertain these thoughts privately. They did not assume she already knew them. They did not affirm their love for her off-handedly on a multitasking busy day.

They took out time. They prepared. They made her the center of their attention and felt their love—and the prospect of her death—in their hearts. Then, in a moment of clarity for them all, they connected at the deepest level with their daughter. The father and mother came to tears. So did Nancy.

"It was wonderful for all of us," he described to me on the third call.

Nancy's parents reached her emotionally, not intellectually. I think of what they did, in the words of Tom Wolfe, as *the right stuff*. I believe that we should all—family members, friends, therapists, doctors, teachers, pastors, and others—aim to develop that ability to the fullest extent possible.

Talking about suicide is challenging to say the least. It's not a panacea. However, it is a vital mission of suicide prevention and a vital mission of this book.

Talk About It

My advice to others to *Talk About It*, directly and head on, did not originate as support and guidance for family members and friends. The concept got its start in a lecture I gave in San Francisco a year after I launched the consultancy. The Northern California Psychiatric Society sponsored the talk. The audience was composed largely of psychiatrists, therapists, counselors, and other mental health professionals. Out of about forty slides I projected on the screen during the presentation, five of them contained a single recurring message: *Talk About It*.

After the lecture I realized I had landed upon a golden principle. I realized that talking about it was something we could all do and teach one another to do—therapists, doctors, nurses, health aides, teachers, police officers, coaches, friends, family members, politicians, and other public figures. Speaking and listening are healing antidotes to shame, stigma, and suicide. Crucially, with a little effort, these skills can be learned.

I never would have written this book without the enthusiastic support and encouragement of so many fellow psychiatrists and psychotherapists. One lunch with a friend and therapist, Robert Solley, stands out as pivotal in my decision-making. At a sunny café at the corner of 18th and Dolores Streets in San Francisco, I told Robert about my idea to compile resources and, in the same

---

Listen. Empathize. Validate.
These constitute a matchless triad.
Then, listen some more.

---

book, to distill the essence of best practices in the screening, assessment, management, and treatment of suicide risk.

We discussed the unique value of a two-part learning and intervention process. In this new model, you assess and manage suicide risk not in the abstract, which is the norm in suicide prevention training, but with the key local resources essential to doing your job well at your fingertips. You learn the *how* of risk assessment and management in combination with the *who*, *what*, *when*, and *where*—names, phone numbers, addresses, and services of life-saving resources and experts—in one book.

The concept had a revolutionary feeling to me—one that could be replicated anywhere in the world—yet I have long since learned to be skeptical of my excitements. It was only when Robert expressed his delight with the idea that I felt emboldened.

"Eli," he said, "I would love to have a book like that!"

Thanks to these heartening words, and those of a dozen other supportive colleagues, I committed to the project and went to work immediately. As envisioned at the lunch with Robert, *Suicide Risk in the Bay Area* is organized precisely to serve as a training manual for suicide risk assessment and management and, in tandem, to provide quick access to more than 300 suicide prevention and treatment services in the Bay Area. The resources include emergency departments, hotlines, mobile crisis units, inpatient units, IOPs, PHPs, clinics, and experts.

Open the book to any page, and you will find helpful resources. In sequential order on the same pages you, will find a training manual for assessment and management as well as resource highlights.

Suicide Risk in the Bay Area, complete with the names and phone numbers of scores of people waiting to hear from you, is an invitation to *Talk About It*. Whether you are a family member, friend, first responder, teacher, doctor, therapist, or other health professional, talking about it is the essence—or at least starting point—of suicide prevention.

Pick up the phone. Make a call. Set up an appointment. You'll be surprised by just how helpful talking about it is.

1

Advocacy

More than anything, this book advocates for open dialogue, discussion, and communication about suicide and suicide risk. This means all people, not just select professionals. No matter where you are or what you do—no matter if you are a teenager, young adult, or mature adult who is experiencing thoughts of suicide; no matter if you are a family member, friend, doctor, therapist, other health professional, or teacher who is concerned about someone—*Talk About It*.

Talk About It. It's at once a simple mandate and a towering challenge. The simplicity is obvious. For someone experiencing suicidal thoughts, it's a mere handful of words to express: "I have been thinking about suicide." For a worried parent, brother, sister, doctor, therapist, or teacher, it's not hard to say, in theory, "Have you had thoughts of ending your life?"

Yet something holds us back. What is it? It's fear combined with thousands of years of entrenched shame and stigma surrounding suicide. Some part of the fear stems from the mistaken belief that talking about it risks planting ideas or opening doors to dangers. But I believe that the lion's share of the fear in those asking, in fact, derives from another source: feelings of helplessness and inadequacy. Not knowing *what to say* or *what to do* engenders avoidance and smothers the simple logic of asking a straightforward question.

Tied to this, there is a common misperception, particularly among health professionals and parents, that you are supposed to respond to a problem—suicide risk—with a solution. Sometimes this is true, no doubt, but do yourself and the person at risk a kind favor: Spend 30 minutes listening. Just listening—nothing else. There is no greater gift you can give to a person suffering emotionally than compassionate listening. When you feel compelled to talk, speak only a few words, and do not speak from fear or authority. Respond with soft, loving words that validate the other's experience and then, quickly, return to listening.

If you feel unskillful at compassionate listening, please know that you are not alone and that the skill can be learned. There are many resources available to you for learning and practicing. These include online programs, videos, audio, workshops, and mindfulness trainings, among others.

So far I have only touched on the role of fear in keeping us from asking simple questions about suicide risk. While recognizing the power of fear, we must not forget the power of shame and stigma. Remember that many world religions have taught sternly for millenia that committing suicide is a sin, an invitation to descend into the depths of Hell. Even an intellect, thinker, and poet as enlightened as Dante advocated this position of the Church in his classic 14th century epic poem *Inferno*. In Circle 7 of Hell, he and Virgil walk through the "Wood of the Self-Murderers." There, the punishment is extreme. Those who commit suicide are transformed into gnarled thorny trees and fed upon, for eternity, by monster-birds called Harpies.

Times have changed, fortunately, but the race is not won. Shame and stigma remain the constant companions of suicide even in daily conversation. There is much advocacy work still to be done. My message is plain: In the face of fear, shame, and stigma, *Talk About It*. Dozens of experts and groups advocate this powerful message, while others train their advocacy on fundraising for research, screening programs, gun safety, hotlines, rapid response teams, legislative lobbying, and barriers at landmark suicide sites like the Golden Gate Bridge.

What unites all these efforts is suicide prevention. All the groups and organizations in this chapter and in this book are dedicated, in their own way, to this singular vital mission. Call them to learn more about the important work they do. Ask them what you can do to support their visions.

SAN FRANCISCO

Mental Health Association of San Francisco (415) 421-2926
Flood Building, 870 Market St #928, San Francisco, CA 94102. www.mentalhealthsf.org. Provides leadership in mental health education, advocacy, research, and policy work. Offers stigma reduction programming, peer support groups, and a group for people who have survived a suicide attempt.

NAMI San Francisco (415) 474-7310 ext. 668
315 Montgomery Street, 2nd Floor, San Francisco, CA 94104. www.namisf.org. A local chapter of this national organization working to advocate for people living with mental illness and to reduce stigma. Provides education, resources, and support for families and those affected by mental illness.

San Francisco Suicide Prevention (415) 984-1900
P.O. Box 191350, San Francisco, CA 94119. www.sfsuicide.org. The nation's oldest suicide hotline and a leader in suicide prevention services and strategies. Provides crisis support hotline, texting, and chat. Offers education in workplaces, churches, organizations, and small groups. Acts as a hub for suicide prevention in San Francisco and collaborates with other organizations on suicide prevention.

Young Minds Advocacy Project (650) 494-4930
901 Mission Street, #105, San Francisco, CA 94103. www.youngmindsadvocacy.org. Works on policy, budgeting, and reform litigation related to mental health services.

EAST BAY

Family Education and Resource Center (510) 746-1700
7200 Bancroft Avenue, Suite 269, Oakland CA 94605. www.askferc.org. An organization providing support to family, friends, and partners of people with serious mental health challenges. Endeavors to reduce stigma surrounding mental health challenges and to educate about appropriate methods of support.

How to Talk About Suicide Risk

Step 1: Ask
Ask the question directly: Are you feeling suicidal? Are you having thoughts of suicide?

Step 2: Listen
If the response is positive, step back and listen. Do not make recommendations. Just listen. Demonstrate that your intention is to listen and understand, not to give solutions or take urgent action.

Step 3: Validate
Validate the person's experience and feelings fully. Validate the human experience of suicidal thoughts and feelings as universal and okay.

Step 4: Keep Listening
If there is silence, you can say, "Tell me more." Or you can ask prompting questions as you would in the discovery of any other type of pain or illness: When did it start? What do you think is the cause? Has it happened before? Is this time the same or worse? What do you think is the most immediate trigger?

Step 5: Assess for Plan, Intent, and Imminence
Again, ask several questions directly: "Do you think you are in fact going to kill yourself? Is it something you think is going to happen? Have you thought about methods or made a suicide plan of any kind? If so, when would it happen? What are the chances that you could die by suicide in the next few days or within the week?"

Step 6: Communicate Value and Hope
Find an earnest, heartfelt way to say that the person matters to you, matters to others, and/or matters to the world. Find hope within yourself about the person and his or her situation first. Then express it.

Step 7: Offer to Help
Ask: "What can I do to help?" When high or imminent risk is not present, you can propose ideas to keep the dialogue going. *Talk About It*

Continued

again soon. Find referrals to mental health professionals. Go to the appointment together. Call a hotline to learn more together about suicide risk. Conduct research that normalizes the experience of suicidal thoughts and feelings as not uncommon in depression and situations of loss, helplessness, and hopelessness. If you are fearful, tell the person. Do not hide it. Ask to call a hotline together to make sure the person is safe and will remain safe.

Step 8: Stay Calm and Connect With Others
Again, if you are concerned that you should do something to potentially save a life, pick up the phone after you *Talk About It* with the person. Now, *Talk About It* with 911, a suicide risk counselor at a hotline or mobile crisis service. You do not need to figure it out alone. There is abundant help available to you. Make a call. Take advantage of the help and resources at your fingertips.

Mental Health Association
of Alameda County (510) 835-5010
954 60th Street, Emeryville, CA 94608. www. mhaac.org. Provides programming concerning early psychosis prevention, support for families of people with mental health challenges, advocation for clients' access to SSI and GA, and a patient rights advocacy program.

NAMI Alameda County (510) 334-7721
954 60th Street, Suite 10, Oakland, CA 94608. www.nami-alamedacounty.org. A local chapter of this national organization working to advocate for people living with mental illness and to reduce stigma. Provides education, resources, and support for families and those affected by mental illness.

NAMI Alameda County South (510) 969-6479
P.O. Box 7302, Fremont, CA 94537. www.namiacs.org. A local chapter of this national organization working to advocate for people living with mental illness and to reduce stigma. Provides education, resources, and support for families and those affected by mental illness.

NAMI Contra Costa County (925) 942-0767
550 Patterson Boulevard, Pleasant Hill, CA 94523. www.namicontracosta.org. A local chapter of this national organization working to advocate for people living with mental illness and to reduce stigma. Provides education, resources, and support for families and those affected by mental illness.

UC Berkeley
You Mean More Group youmeanmore@gmail.com
UC Berkeley Campus, Berkeley, CA. www.youmeanmore.wordpress.com. A suicide prevention group for UC Berkeley students endeavoring to raise awareness and reduce stigma around mental health conditions and suicide. You Mean More organizes the annual UC Berkeley Suicide Prevention Walk, movie nights, and mental health monologue events.

NORTH BAY

The Bridge Rail Foundation info@bridgerail.org
3020 Bridgeway #179, Sausalito, CA 94965. www.bridgerail.org. An advocacy organization endeavoring to end suicide on the Golden Gate Bridge by building a safety net around the bridge.

Marin Teen Mental Health Board (415) 272-5123
317 Scenic Road, Fairfax, CA 94930. john@iheartcasey.com. A peer- support group endeavoring to train and educate Marin County high school students and their parents about suicide and depression. Founded and facilitated by several Marin high school students and an adult supervisor as a response to several suicides of Marin youth.

NAMI Marin County (415) 444-0480
555 Northgate Drive, #280, San Rafael, CA 94903. www.namimarin.org. A local chapter of this national organization dedicated to improving the lives of individuals and families living with mental illness, through advocacy, education, and support.

Core Components of Assessment & Management

- Screening
- Assessment
- Risk Formulation
- Management
- Treatment

NAMI Solano County (707) 422-7792

P.O. Box 3334, Fairfield, CA 94533. www.namisolanocounty.org. A local chapter of this national organization working to advocate for people living with mental illness and to reduce stigma. Provides education, resources, and support for families and those affected by mental illness. Serves Solano and Napa Counties.

NAMI Sonoma County (707) 527-6655

182 Farmers Lane, Suite 202, Santa Rosa, CA 95405. www.namiso-co.org. A local chapter of this national organization working to advocate for people living with mental illness and to reduce stigma. Provides education, resources, and support for families and those affected by mental illness.

North Bay Suicide Prevention Project (415) 499-1193 Ext. 3004

555 Northgate Drive, San Rafael, CA 94903. www.fsamarin.org. A collaborative between the Family Services Agency of Marin and the 5 counties of the North Bay. Provides hotline services to each county and offers a variety of trainings, including ASIST, QPR, safeTALK, and AMSR. This project also works in collaboration with other suicide prevention projects and organizations in the Bay Area to design effective prevention strategies.

PENINSULA

Kara (650) 321-5272

457 Kingsley Avenue, Palo Alto, CA 94301. www.kara-grief.org. A nonprofit organization providing grief support to children, teens, families and adults. Offers presentations and workshops on subjects including personal death awareness, how to talk to childen about death, and cultivating compassionate presence to community organizations like faith groups, senior groups, schools, and the general public.

NAMI San Mateo County (650) 638-0800

1650 Borel Place, Suite 130, San Mateo, CA 94010. www.namisanmateo.org. A local chapter of the national organization. Offers peer-support groups, advocacy, and family support groups as well as trainings on mental health support.

Project Safety Net (650) 463-4928

4000 Middlefield Road, Palo Alto, CA 94306. www.psnpaloalto.com. A coalition of community members and residents of the Palo Alto area. Plans suicide intervention, prevention, and education opportunities in the community. Formed in response to a growing need after 5 young people in the district completed suicide.

San Mateo County Behavioral Health and Recovery Services Division (650) 638-0800

1650 Borel Place, Suite 130, San Mateo, CA 94010. www.namisanmateo.org. A local chapter of the national organization. Offers peer-support groups, advocacy, and family support groups as well as trainings on mental health support.

SOUTH BAY

Law Foundation of Silicon Valley Mental Health Advocacy Project (408) 293-4790

152 North Third Street, 3rd Floor. San Jose, CA 95112. www.lawfoundation.org. An advocacy project that provides legal assistance

to people who identify as having a mental health or developmental disability. Advocates for personal rights, poverty prevention, housing rights, and patient rights.

NAMI Santa Clara County (408) 453-0400

1150 S. Bascom Avenue, Suite 24, San Jose, CA 95128. Monday to Friday: 10:00 a.m to 2:00 a.m. www.namisantaclara.org. A local chapter of the national organization. Offers peer-support groups, advocacy, and family support groups as well as trainings on mental health support.

BAY AREA

Bay Area Suicide and Crisis Intervention Alliance (BASCIA)

www.bascia.org. An alliance of suicide prevention agencies. Member organizations offer a range of services including crisis support and suicide prevention education. BASCIA is comprised of Crisis Support Services of Alameda County, Contra Costa Crisis Center, Family Services Agency of Marin, San Francisco Suicide Prevention, San Mateo County's StarVista Crisis Intervention and Suicide Prevention Program, and The BridgeRail Foundation. Offers online resources, statewide advocacy, and support for new suicide prevention programs.

Greater San Francisco Bay Area Chapter of the
American Foundation for Suicide Prevention (707) 968-7563

2471 Solano Avenue, Suite 114, Napa, CA 94558. sfbayarea@afsp. org. Local chapter of this national organization. Funds research, creates educational programs, advocates for public policy, and supports survivors of suicide loss. This local chapter hosts a wide variety of activities throughout the region ranging from outreach and education events, to presentations and conferences, to public events like the Out of the Darkness Walks each Fall and Spring and the International Survivors of Suicide Loss Day Conference each November.

Common Suicide Risk Screening Questions

- Have you ever had thoughts that you'd rather be dead?
- Have you ever had suicidal thoughts?
- Sometimes people feel so depressed/bad/low that they have thoughts of ending their own lives. Has that happened to you?
- Have you recently been feeling hopeless?
- Have you recently had thoughts that you'd rather be dead?
- Have you recently felt that you or your family would be better off if you were dead?
- Have you recently had thoughts of killing yourself?
- Have you had these thoughts today? Yesterday?
- Have you ever made a suicide attempt?
- Have you ever made a plan to kill yourself?
- Have you been having any thoughts of suicide at all, even a little?

Northern California Psychiatric Society (415) 334-2418
77 Van Ness Avenue, Suite 101, #2022, San Francisco, CA 94102. www.ncps.org. Promotes the effectiveness of psychiatry through advocacy, professional education, and community-building.

CALIFORNIA

California Mental Health
Service Authority (CalMHSA) (916) 859-4806
An organization endeavoring to develop and implement strategies and programs for suicide prevention and mental health support.

NATIONAL

American Association of Suicidology (202) 237-2280
5221 Wisconsin Avenue, NW, Washington, DC 20015. www.suicidolgy.org. A national association dedicated to understanding and

Evidence-Based Suicide Prevention Interventions

- Means restriction
- Physician education
- Screening
- Pharmacotherapy
- Psychotherapy

preventing suicide. Seeks to advance Suicidology as a science and to research and publicly share accurate information on suicidal behaviors and high quality suicide prevention.

American Foundation for Suicide Prevention (AFSP) 1-888-333-AFSP

www.afsp.org. A national organization working to produce leadership, research, prevention programming, community education tools, and a fundraiser walk called "Out of the Darkness," available in many cities across the United States. 67 chapters are based throughout the nation, which host local programs and events.

Center for the Prevention of Suicide (215) 898-4102

3535 Market Street, Room 2032, Philadelphia, PA, 19104. www.med.upenn.edu/suicide. A research center based out of the University of Pennsylvania. Endeavors to develop innovative Cognitive Therapy treatments for the prevention of suicide that can be disseminated into local settings and pre-existing programs around the country. Works toward real-world solutions for patients.

The Jed Foundation (212) 647-7544

6 East 39th Street, Suite 1204, New York, NY 10016. www.jedfoundation.org. A national organization dedicated to promoting emotional health and preventing suicide among college and university students. Collaborates with mtvU on halfofus.com, which uses sto-

ries of students and high-profile artists to increase awareness about mental health problems and the importance of getting help. Runs the ULifeline.org online mental health support network.

National Alliance on Mental Illness (NAMI) (703) 524-7600

www.nami.org. A national organization working to advocate for people living with mental illness and to reduce stigma. Local chapters can be found around the Bay Area.

Suicide Prevention Resource Center 1-877-GET-SPRC

www.sprc.org. A national organization providing organizational support, partnerships building, training, technical assistance, resources, and a best practices registry to support suicide prevention initiatives.

2

Broad-Based Suicide Prevention

The organizations contained in this chapter are an excellent starting point for family members, friends, health professionals, teachers, and other professionals interested in building their skills in suicide prevention and expanding their knowledge base of local and national resources. Although the organizations are categorized by geographic region, you should feel free to contact any or all of them for information and guidance, no matter where you live or work. The staff are happy to answer your questions. They are happy to coach you. They will gladly link you to other resources that better fit your needs.

"Broad-based" signifies that these organizations do not have a single area of focus, such as crisis management or triage. Instead, they are multifaceted in their suicide prevention activities and services. For example, the North Bay Suicide Prevention Project operates a 24/7 crisis line and offers sliding-scale grief counseling. Additionally, the project provides professional, peer, and family member trainings in prevention. One modality the North Bay Suicide Prevention Project employs in its trainings is QPR: Question, Persuade, Refer. Staff and volunteers educate others in what is called the "Chain of Survival": Early recognition of warning signs >> question >> intervention and referral >> professional assessment and treatment.

North Bay Suicide Prevention and other broad-based organizations often rely on another comprehensive national training program called Applied Suicide Intervention Skills Training (ASIST). The ASIST modality teaches suicide prevention "first aid" to mental health professionals as well as to a wide network of "gatekeepers"—that is, community members in prime positions to be the first to notice warning signs. Gatekeepers include physicians, nurses, dieticians, teachers, guidance counselors, sports coaches, professional coaches, first responders, clergy, family, and friends, among others. These individuals are on the front lines and, with basic education, can learn to detect warning signs, ask, and intervene effectively.

Beyond hotlines, grief counseling, and in-person trainings, broad-based suicide prevention organizations offer other valuable information and services, including:

- Libraries, publications, and newsletters
- Guidance in creating suicide prevention programs
- Suicide-related research results and statistics
- Funding sources for suicide-related research
- Support groups, work groups, and outreach projects
- Online trainings and webinars
- Public lectures and awareness campaigns
- Media and marketing advice

These and other prevention organizations advocate a central premise: basic suicide prevention is a form of psychiatric "CPR" that can be learned by anyone. Observing, asking, and intervening is as straightforward and mechanical as checking an unconscious person's pulse and, when absent, applying chest compressions and rescue breathing.

Do not hesitate to call these organizations. Pick up the phone and begin a dialogue. If you feel the first organization you contact does not successfully answer your questions or meet your needs, reach out to another. Talking about it is the true starting point for improving your skills and level of confidence in helping someone with potential suicide risk.

BAY AREA

Bay Area Suicide and Crisis Intervention Alliance (BASCIA)

www.bascia.org. An alliance of suicide prevention agencies. Member organizations offer a range of services including crisis support and suicide prevention education. BASCIA is comprised of Crisis Support Services of Alameda County, Contra Costa Crisis Center, Family Services Agency of Marin, San Francisco Suicide Prevention, San Mateo County's StarVista Crisis Intervention and Suicide Prevention Program, and The BridgeRail Foundation. Offers online resources, statewide advocacy, and support for new suicide prevention programs.

Greater San Francisco Bay Area Chapter of the
American Foundation for Suicide Prevention (707) 968-7563

2471 Solano Avenue, Suite 114, Napa, CA 94558. www.afsp.org. Local chapter of this national organization. Funds research, creates educational programs, advocates for public policy, and supports survivors of suicide loss. This local chapter hosts a wide variety of activities throughout the region ranging from outreach and education events, to presentations and conferences, to public events like the Out of the Darkness Walks each Fall and Spring and the International Survivors of Suicide Loss Day Conference each November.

SAN FRANCISCO

San Francisco Suicide Prevention (415) 984-1900

P.O. Box 191350, San Francisco, CA 94119. www.sfsuicide.org. The nation's oldest suicide hotline and a leader in suicide prevention services and strategies. Provides crisis support hotline, texting, and chat. Offers education in workplaces, churches, organizations, and small groups. Support groups are available for people who have survived a suicide attempt. Risk reduction programs are available for youth. Acts as a hub for suicide prevention in San Francisco and collaborates with other organizations on suicide prevention.

Personal Calling and Mission: Youth Suicide Risk

Although it was my mother, not my child, who died by suicide, my passion is suicide prevention in adolescents and young adults. Suicide is always tragic, but youth suicide is something uniquely grievous, heartrending, and patently wrong in our society.

As this book is being published, I am launching an initiative called the "Youth Suicide Risk Research Project." The purpose of this initiative is to investigate and document evidence-based strategies for identifying and treating youth suicide risk.

Read more about youth suicide prevention in the Introduction to Chapter 11, "Adolescent and Youth Services."

Sign up for news on the Youth Suicide Risk Research Project under "Mental Health Compass" on the Merritt Mental Health website. To share ideas or collaborate in the project, please email info@merrittmentalhealth.com.

Suicide Prevention Team
at the SFVA Medical Center (415) 221-4810

4150 Clement Street, San Francisco, CA 94121. www.sanfrancisco. va.gov. A program acting as part of a VA national strategy to address the problem of suicidality in the vetran population. Offers a wide range of administrative, clinical, educational, and community outreach activities focused on suicide prevention. Offers consultation and support to medical and mental health providers across the San Francisco VA system to enhance the quality of care offered to at-risk patients.

NORTH BAY

Marin Teen Mental Health Board (415) 272-5123

317 Scenic Road, Fairfax CA 94930. john@iheartcasey.com. A peer-support group endeavoring to train and educate Marin county high school students and their parents about suicide and depression. Founded and facilitated by several Marin high school students and an adult supervisor as a response to several suicides of Marin youth.

North Bay
Suicide Prevention Project (415) 499-1193 Ext. 3004
555 Northgate Drive, San Rafael, CA 94903. www.fsamarin.org. A collaborative between the Family Services Agency of Marin and the 5 counties of the North Bay. Provides hotline services to each county and offers a variety of trainings, including ASIST, QPR, safeTALK, and AMSR. This project also works in collaboration with other suicide prevention projects and organizations in the Bay Area to design effective prevention strategies.

PENINSULA

Project Safety Net (650) 463-4928
4000 Middlefield Road, Palo Alto, CA 94306. www.psnpaloalto.com. A coalition of community members and residents of the Palo Alto area. Plans suicide intervention, prevention and education opportunities in the community. Formed in response to a growing need after 5 young people in the district completed suicide.

NATIONAL

American Association of Suicidology (202) 237-2280
5221 Wisconsin Avenue, NW, Washington, DC 20015. www.suicidology.org. A national association dedicated to understanding and preventing suicide. Seeks to advance Suicidology as a science and to research and publicly share accurate information on suicidal behaviors and high quality suicide prevention.

American Foundation for Suicide Prevention 1-888-333-2377
120 Wall Street, 29th Floor, New York, NY 10005. www.afsp.org. A national suicide prevention organization that funds research, creates educational programs, advocates for public policy, and supports survivors of suicide loss. 67 chapters are based throughout the nation, which host local programs and events.

When to Assess for Suicide Risk

- When there is initial concern
- At intake appointments
- When suicidal thoughts or feelings are mentioned or discovered
- After suicidal behaviors
- When symptoms of depression or other conditions worsen
- Upon a sudden, dramatic improvement in mood or functioning (it is well-documented that a decision to commit suicide may generate relief from hopelessness and abrupt mood improvement)
- After significant interpersonal loss or psychosocial stressors such as job loss, divorce, or onset of physical illness
- After psychiatric hospitalizations

The Jed Foundation (212) 647-7544
6 East 39th Street, Suite 1204, New York, NY 10016. www.jedfoundation.org. A national organization dedicated to promoting emotional health and preventing suicide among college and university students. Collaborates with the public and leaders in higher education, mental health, and research to produce and advance initiatives that promote awareness and understanding, foster help-seeking, and raise the importance of suicide prevention solutions.

Center for the Prevention of Suicide (215) 898-4102
3535 Market Street, Room 2032, Philadelphia, PA, 19104. www.med.upenn.edu/suicide. A research center based out of the University of Pennsylvania. Endeavors to develop innovative Cognitive Therapy treatments for the prevention of suicide that can be disseminated into local settings and pre-existing programs around the country. Works toward real-world solutions for patients.

Sources of Strength
Suicide Prevention Program (701) 471-7183
www.sourcesofstrength.org. A national suicide prevention program that trains peers and adults to lead support groups in high

schools. Provides several groups across the Bay Area. Endeavors to reduce stigma surrounding suicide.

Suicide Awareness Voices of Education (SAVE) (952) 946-7998 www.save.org. Provides education, school-based programs, a speaker's bureau, professional trainings, public awareness campaigns, and support groups on suicide prevention.

3

Hotlines

In the present day suicide prevention hotlines exist in most counties and major cities in the United States. Unknown to most Bay Area residents, however, San Francisco played a transformative role in the early history of 24-hour hotlines. In 1961 an activist teacher turned Anglican priest, Bernard Mayes, set up the nation's first hotline in the Tenderloin District.

Alarmed upon learning of San Francisco's high suicide rate, Mayes, who a decade later became the founding chairman of National Public Radio, initiated a grassroots prevention campaign, replete with flyers and advertisements posted on billboards and city buses. The organization he founded, San Francisco Suicide Prevention, soon adopted a catchy motto: "Thinking of ending it all? Call Bruce, PR1-0450, San Francisco Suicide Prevention."

Today San Francisco Suicide Prevention (SFSP) still operates the 24-hour crisis line Mayes founded and is regarded as a beacon in the field. A single red phone rang in 1961, and, half a century later, a dozen of them ring nearly 200 times a day at the San Francisco headquarters. SFSP employs 10 staff members, but its lifeblood is 100 volunteers who undergo extensive training and listen and guide callers 24/7.

"I did feel that what was really needed was a compassionate ear, someone to talk to," Mayes told the San Francisco Chronicle in

2012. "It occurred to me that we had to have some kind of service which would offer unconditional listening, and that I would be this anonymous ear."

Eve Meyer, SFSP's current Executive Director, cites statistics demonstrating that the city's suicide rate is less than half what it was when the agency was founded.

Mayes gave San Francisco citizens a confidential dependable place to *Talk About It*. Today SFPS operates its many phone lines and offers free trainings to law enforcement, health professionals, and schools. Anyone can call and make inquiries, not just individuals with suicidal thoughts and feelings. SFSP educates and guides the general public, including family members, friends, teachers, nurses, doctors, and other health professionals.

Call this crisis service, or any of the two dozen other Bay Area and national hotlines listed in this chapter, 24 hours per day. Whatever your question, ask it. Whatever your concern, discuss it. Whatever's on your mind, you are sure to find a friendly, compassionate person on the other end of the phone line interested in helping.

CALIFORNIA

California Youth Crisis Line 1-800-843-5200

Offers conference calls to guardians, among other regular hotline services.

SAN FRANCISCO

Center for Elderly Suicide Prevention 1-800-971-0016

Serves seniors, their caregivers, and their advocates. The number above connects to the Center's 24/7 friendship line.

Huckleberry Youth House Crisis
24-Hour Hotline (415) 621-2929

Serves children and adolescents, ages 1-17. Parents, caretakers, and mental health providers are also encouraged to call.

Mental Health Peer-Run Warm Line 1-855-845-7415

Offers peer support to those with mental health conditions and suicidal ideation.

San Francisco 24-Hour Access Helpline (415) 255-3737

Provided by San Francisco's Community Behavioral Health Services.

San Francisco Suicide Prevention (415) 781-0500

The nation's oldest suicide hotline. See featured resource of the same name. Access lines are available for specific needs:
Text Message Access Text "MYLIFE" to 741741
HIV Nightline (415) 434-2437
Linea de Apoyo (415) 989-5212
Drug Information Line (415) 362-3400
Relapse Line (415) 834-1144
TTY (415) 227-0245

Trans Lifeline (877) 565-8860

Hours vary. A hotline run by transgender people for transgender people.

Suicidal Ideation: Frequency, Duration, and Intensity

- Over the past few days how often have you thought about suicide? Every hour, 4-5 times per day, twice per day, once per day?
- When suicidal thoughts come into your mind, how long do they last? Does a thought stay with you for 30-45 minutes, 5 minutes, 1 minute, a few seconds?
- How intense have the suicidal thoughts been? Would you say that they are thoughts that feel weak, somewhat strong, strong, or very strong?

EAST BAY

Contra Costa Crisis Center 1-800-833-2900
County-run hotline. TTD/TTY: (925) 938-0725

Crisis Support Services of Alameda County 1-800-309-2131
County-run hotline.

NORTH BAY

Marin County Crisis Line (415) 499-1100
County-run hotline.

North Bay Suicide Prevention 1-855-587-6373
North Bay-wide hotline facilitated by Family Services Agency of Marin, a community center, and the four counties of the North Bay.

PENINSULA

Child & Adolescent Hotline and Prevention Program (650) 567-5437
Star Vista-run hotline serving children, adolescents, and their families. Accepts calls and texts.

Línea de Crisis 1-800-303-7432
Star Vista-run hotline serving Spanish speakers in San Mateo County.

Star Vista Crisis Line (650) 579-0350
San Mateo County-run suicide prevention and mental health crisis line.

SOUTH BAY

Bill Wilson Center Crisis Line (408) 850-6125
Provides crisis line for all ages. Bill Wilson Center works primarily with youth and adolescents.

Chat 4 Teens www.billwilsoncenter.org
www.billwilsoncenter.org/services/all/teens.html. Monday to Friday: 5 p.m. to 9 p.m. Provides live online chat support for teenagers residing in Santa Clara County. A safe and anonymous service offering space for venting, connecting, and gaining information about community resources. This service is provided by Bill Willson Center.

Suicide and Crisis Services
of Santa Clara County 1-855-278-4204
County-run hotline.

International Suicide Statistics

- Over 800,000 people die due to suicide each year, with many more who attempt suicide.
- On average, one person dies by suicide every 40 seconds somewhere in the world.
- In 2012, suicide was the second leading cause of death among 15-to-29-year-olds.
- Suicide accounted for 1.4% of all deaths worldwide, making it the 15th leading cause of death in 2012.
- Global suicide rates have increased 60% in the past 45 years.

World Health Organization, 2012

NATIONAL

Crisis Text Line Text "START" to 741741
Provides text message crisis support.

Lifeline Crisis Chat www.suicidepreventionlifeline.org
Offers live Internet chat to help reduce stress and increase feelings of empowerment.

Red Nacional de Prevención del Suicidio 1-877-784-2432
National hotline for Spanish-language speakers.

NAMI Information Hotline 1-800-950-6264
Facilitated by the National Alliance on Mental Illness (NAMI). In addition to regular hotline services, NAMI offers information on mental illness, legal resources, and peer support.

National S.A.F.E Alternatives Hotline 1-800-366-8288
Committed to helping those with self-injurous behavior.

National Suicide Prevention Lifeline 1-800-273-8255
Connects callers with local services.

4

Mobile Crisis Services

Mobile Crisis is specifically meant to intervene in behavioral crises, not medical emergencies. This service, despite its slightly misleading designation "crisis," is in fact for *non-emergencies*—that is, behavioral problems or concerns that can wait patiently for at least one hour, often two or three hours, to be attended to. It is worth underscoring the fundamental principle that for any life-threatening circumstance, immediately call 911:

- If there is imminent risk of loss of life or limb, of any kind, call 911.
- If a dangerous weapon is involved, call 911.
- If someone is severely injured or gravely ill, call 911.

Many mobile crisis units operate phone and field services during restricted hours. You might call and encounter a delay. You might be rolled over to a voicemail system and asked to leave a message. Therefore, if you are uncertain of the degree of dangerousness involved, call 911. Do not delay.

The distinction between behavioral crisis and medical emergency is vital. Everyone concerned about potential suicide risk should take the time to understand it. In a *crisis*, you perceive an urgent need for assistance. In a *medical emergency*, you are concerned about immediate death or serious injury. In the case of suicide risk, the following situations are medical emergencies that should prompt a call to 911:

- A serious medication or drug overdose
- A serious suicide threat involving the imminent use of a gun or other dangerous weapon
- An imminent threat to jump
- Any serious intent to die by suicide imminently

The operative word in a psychiatric medical emergency is *imminent*. If there is an imminent risk of suicide, call 911.

Hence, what is the value of a mobile crisis service? When should a doctor, therapist, or family member call this service instead of 911? These are examples of circumstances where mobile crisis intervention is indicated:

- You perceive some degree of suicide risk, but not imminent risk. Time is not of the essence. You wish for guidance, perhaps a phone or field assessment, and you have time to make the call, discuss the situation, and follow the directions of the mobile crisis clinician aiding you.
- An acute risk of suicide occurred but has passed. The individual is currently safe. You remain worried and wish for assessment, guidance, or intervention.
- There is no medical emergency. Yet the person with potential suicide risk cannot or will not seek professional help. Call mobile crisis for guidance and a possible field visit.

Mobile crisis services in the Bay Area are vastly different from one another. Some welcome phone calls. Some do not. Some operate

24/7. Others do not. Some see adolescents. Others do not. A wise course of action, whenever time allows, is to call your local suicide hotline or mobile crisis service—or both—and ask questions. Ask and keep asking until you feel confident you understand your local resources and the procedures they follow to help you.

One disadvantage of mobile crisis is the considerable time it requires for the professionals to arrive on the scene of a crisis, as compared to police and ambulance services. One advantage, however, is that mobile crisis stays longer and is more comprehensive in its assessment and management of suicide risk. Mobile crisis strives to resolve crises in the field. Many operate under the specific mandate to *avoid hospitalization* whenever possible. Their mission is to intervene, stabilize, and treat in the *least restrictive environment*. Mobile crisis clinicians are mental health experts. They are skilled at using a client's strengths and natural supports to resolve the immediate crisis.

Another significant advantage of a mobile crisis organization is the ongoing guidance, referrals, and support many provide once the crisis has passed. Some offer 30-day continuing stabilization and counseling to clients and family members. Often they provide care coordination, transitions to intensive outpatient programs, and referrals to psychotherapists and psychiatrists. When hospitalization is necessary, some mobile crisis services provide discharge and aftercare planning to smooth the transition back home and into outpatient care.

No matter whether you are a health professional, friend, or family member, if you are worried about suicide risk in any way, become familiar with your local mobile crisis service. Know the phone number. Become informed. Become prepared. Remember that the services provided vary widely by organization, so call and ask questions about procedures and protocols until you are confident you understand what to do in a crisis.

SAN FRANCISCO

Comprehensive Child Crisis Service (415) 970-3800
www.sfdph.org. 24/7. A crisis intervention service for children and adolescents in San Francisco. Provides 30 days of ongoing stabilization and crisis management for approved clients.

Mobile Crisis Treatment Team (415) 970-4000
www.sfdph.org. Monday to Friday: 8:30 a.m. to 11 p.m.; Saturday: 12 p.m. to 8 p.m. Serves adults in San Franscico. While phones stay open for all hours listed above, the Mobile Crisis Treatment Team (MCTT) usually conducts their last in-person visit one hour before close: 10 p.m. from Monday to Friday and 7 p.m. on Sat. Non-crisis calls made in this final hour will be addressed the following day. Provides 30 days of ongoing stabilization and crisis management for approved clients.

San Francisco Homeless
Outreach Team (SFHOT) (415) 241-1184
50 Ivy Street, SF, CA 94102. www.catsinc.org. Provides short-term crisis stabilization in the community, case management, outreach, warm hand-offs between street involved people and hospitals, and helps to support people's location of a shelter/SRO. Call 311 and ask for SFHOT.

EAST BAY

Berkeley Mental Health Mobile Crisis Team (510) 981-5900
www.ci.berkeley.ca.us. 11:30 a.m. to 10:00 p.m., 7 days per week and all holidays. Serves residents of Berkeley and Albany. For immediate access to the Mobile Crisis Team during working hours, call the Berkeley Police Department's non-emergency number at (510) 981-5900 and ask to speak to a mental health worker. For 24-hour mental health crisis assistance by phone, call Crisis Services of Alameda County at (800) 309-2131.

Comprehensive Child Crisis Service

This crisis service in San Francisco is widely praised for its efficiency, thoroughness, and soft touch when it comes to youth and their families. It is an exemplar of behavioral crisis intervention worthy of emulation by mental health professionals, clinics, and agencies nationwide.

Comprehensive Child Crisis is timely. It conducts careful assessments of clients and the "villages" of people surrounding them—teachers, peers, family members, and neighbors. Its dedicated aim is crisis stabilization, where possible without hospitalization. It allows walk-ins to its main office. It operates, in partnership with a residential treatment center, a short-term "crisis stabilization unit," providing clients and their families immediate access to a safe containing environment.

The clinicians at Child Crisis realize the job is not done once they depart the home or school where they crisis took place. They understand the power of intervention to bring families together and to heal. Their goal in a field-based intervention is to open communication and initiate change. They stick with the family over time. They follow up. They form relationships. They guide, direct, and connect, ushering the family towards maximum health.

When hospitalization is necessary, the service additionally provides a specialized "discharge planner" to ensure a smooth transition to outpatient clinicians and programs. Understanding the real needs of families in distress, Comprehensive Child Crisis further offers a 30-day intensive case management program. When necessary, they follow-up with families and manage evolving challenges on a daily basis.

Take as one example a phone call to Child Crisis by the mother of a 15-year-old who has said openly that life is not worth living—he intends to hang himself. At the moment, he is in his room listening to music. His face is long and pained. The music heard through the door is solemn and downcast. His grades are poor. Recently, a group of friends rejected him. He feels hopeless he'll ever recover. His family is frightened he'll take his own life.

The mother calls 415-970-3800. First, the clinician on duty ascertains that there is no immediate threat to his life. Has he overdosed?

Continued

Does he have a gun? Is he hanging himself presently? The clinician obtains more history and decides to send a mobile crisis unit to the house to assess, stabilize, and plan.

A team of two arrives at the house thirty minutes later. They speak to the family and again confirm the adolescent's current safety. They obtain a detailed mental health and risk history. Next, they speak to the adolescent. By way of careful listening, they open communication and assess suicide risk. If risk has dissipated, they formulate an outpatient plan that includes follow-up at the Child Crisis office in San Francisco. If there is agitation, hopelessness, and ongoing moderate to high suicide risk, they transport to the crisis stabilization unit for up to 24 hours of monitoring. There, clinicians continue therapeutic intervention and treatment planning.

Comprehensive Child Crisis does not ignore the family. They educate the family. They coach the family. They teach assessment techniques, empathic listening, and coping skills. They link the adolescent and family to appropriate outpatient services and programs. They invite some clients with Medi-Cal to enroll in the service's 30-day Crisis Stabilization Program. For all families, they strive to restore health through individualized treatment planning and therapeutic connection to family, friends, faith communities, cultural communities, and self-help groups.

Vitally, the crisis clinicians develop a treatment plan that incorporates the family *over the long term*. Comprehensive Child Crisis Service of San Francisco earns its designation "comprehensive" on a daily basis. Widely respected in San Francisco, the service deserves to be studied as a model of excellence nationwide, even worldwide.

Contra Costa County Mobile Crisis Team 911

www.cchealth.org. Serves the elderly in Contra Costa County. Although little information is available on this team, the Contra Costa Regional Medical Center suggests that the best mobile services for Contra Costa adults can be accessed by dialing 911. Children and adolescents can access mobile crisis services by calling Seneca at (877) 411-1089.

North County Mobile Crisis Team (800) 491-9099

Monday to Friday: 10 a.m. to 7 p.m. Serves adults in Alameda County. Child and adolescent cases are diverted to the nearest Emergency Department. The above number is a direct line to ACCESS, Alameda County's 24-hour hub for behavioral health assistance, which evaluates each situation to see if Mobile Crisis Services are the best solution.

Seneca Mobile Response Team (877) 441-1089

www.senecaofa.org/crisis. 11:00 a.m. to 9:00 p.m., 7 days per week. 24-hour phone support. Serves youth and families in Alameda and Contra Costa Counties. If deemed necessary, the MRT invite youth and families into a 20-to-30-day program, which provides general support and mental health services. The Team may also enter youth and family into Seneca's Short-Term Assessment of Resources and Treatment (START) program, which offers resources and treatment including family therapy, psychiatry, and support groups.

NORTH BAY

Crisis, Assessment, Prevention, and Education (CAPE) Team (707) 565-3542

www.sonoma-county.org. A county mental health service providing mobile outreach and assessments. Offers trainings for peers and parents on suicide prevention and mental health awareness.

Exodus Solano Mobile Crisis Team (707) 784-2080

2101 Courage Drive, Fairfield, CA 94533. www.exodusrecovery-inc.com. 24/7. A crisis intervention service for residents of Solano County. Offers immediate crisis evaluations and crisis stabilization services in the community and at the Fairfield Crisis Stabilization Unit.

Common Crisis Services

- Crisis intervention
- Crisis de-escalation and stabilization
- Conflict resolution
- Telephone risk assessment and crisis counseling
- Family education, guidance, and support
- Advice to health professionals
- Field visits to homes, schools, and other community settings
- Emergency medication management
- Referrals and linkage to services
- Involuntary hospitalization by California state law 5150
- Safety and prevention planning
- Follow-up care and case management

Napa County Crisis Unit (707) 253-4711

www.countyofnapa.org. Monday to Friday: 7 am to 6 pm. Serves residents of Napa County. Although the mobile team's hours are limited, the above number is an active 24/7 crisis line staffed by emergency response workers. The mobile team is a service of Napa County Crisis Unit, which also offers walk-in evaluations at 2344 Old Sonoma Road, Bldg. D, Napa, CA 94559.

Sonoma County Mobile Support Team (707) 565-6900

www.sonoma-county.org. Hours vary. A crisis intervention service that works in collaboration with the police to serve residents of Sonoma County. Operates during peak activity hours and days as informed by ongoing data review and coordination with law enforcement agencies. The team is staffed by licensed mental health clinicians, certified substance abuse specialists, post-graduate registered interns, mental health consumers, and family members. The team intentionally works to connect patients with appropriate resources.

PENINSULA

Mateo Lodge (650) 368-3178

www.mateolodge.org. An appointment-based mobile crisis assistance service for adults in San Mateo County. Provides evaluations, counseling, and entry into the county mental health system and its resources for situations in the home as well as the homeless.

SOUTH BAY

EMQ Families First Mobile Crisis Program (408) 379-9085

251 Llewellyn Avenue, Campbell, CA 95008. www.emqff.org. 24/7. A crisis intervention service for children and adolescents in Santa Clara County. EMQ Families First Crisis Stabilization Unit can be reached at (408) 364-4083.

5

Emergency Departments

Emergency departments may seem to be straightforward medical entities requiring little further elaboration beyond naming them and providing an accompanying address and telephone number. In truth, from the psychiatric perspective, a great transformation has come over hospital emergency services in the past two decades. Chiefly, what has changed is access to inpatient psychiatric beds. There has been a considerable contraction of beds and a tightening of reimbursement from government and commercial insurance since the 1980s, all of which translates into a diminished ability of emergency department clinical staff to hospitalize patients who present with suicide risk.

This is not to say that emergency departments are recklessly turning away patients at risk of death who need to be hospitalized. It means the bar of risk has been raised. Whereas in the 1980s suicidal thoughts may have been a sufficient enough concern to prompt hospitalization for several days, the standard today has moved towards a medico-legal foundation. Typically, the patient must meet criteria for an involuntary commitment, even if he or she is admitted voluntarily.

In California this standard is set by section 5150 of the Lanterman-Petris-Short Act authorizing a qualified clinician or law enforcement official to involuntarily confine a person deemed to be at risk of suicide for up to three days of observation. Surprisingly, state law does not define risk. It leaves the interpretation and stratification of risk open to the judgment of the clinician or officer.

What has evolved in California in light of this absence of clear legal criteria for hospitalization is the *standard of imminence*. Suicidal ideation is no longer considered adequate grounds for hospitalization. Neither is an indistinct plan to commit suicide or even future intent based on depressing contingencies such as possible coming job loss, relationship break-up, divorce, or other significant life dislocations.

The standard of imminence means that a person has a plan, clear intent, and the risk of death is imminent. *Imminence* itself is another yardstick open to variable interpretation. Does imminent risk of suicide denote risk of death within hours, days, or weeks? In my consultations with forensic psychiatrists and emergency department directors in the Bay Area, consensus seemed to emerge solidly around days as the touchstone, not hours or weeks.

If a clinician evaluating a patient in an emergency department (ED) concludes that there is a reasonable probability of death by suicide within one, two, or three days, the clinician is expected, by legal standard of care, to issue a 5150 involuntary hold and hospitalize.

"No imminence, no hospitalization" is one way to think of today's climate for psychiatric hospitalization for suicide risk in the San Francisco Bay Area.

Family members, friends, psychiatrists, therapists, teachers, and other professionals should be aware of this state of affairs before driving to the ED or recommending this course of action. Especially psychiatrists and therapists must recognize that their training, expertise, and immediate concerns count for little once one of their patients arrives at the doors of the department. Clinicians there will make their own assessment. Do not anticipate that because you have declared suicide risk to be present that your patient will be hospitalized. Chances are good and growing, it seems, that your patient will in fact not be hospitalized. Before directing patients and family members to the ED, carefully assess for ideation, plan, intent, and imminence.

It is perfectly okay for a patient to go to the ED for an assessment. Expert opinion is worth its weight in gold. It can save lives.

It can reduce extreme worry in patients, family members, friends, and outpatient clinicians. It can mark a turning point in a person's life and willingness to seek psychiatric care. My caveat relates only to what you expect to happen: *Do not go to the ED expecting a person with suicide risk to be hospitalized.*

In this chapter you will notice a distinction between standard EDs and EDs with Psychiatric Emergency Service (PES) units. A PES is a specialized psychiatric emergency department, typically located adjacent to a medical emergency department. What you should know is that these units are staffed entirely by nurses, doctors, and aides who specialize in psychiatry and psychiatric emergencies. Additionally, they are better equipped than standard EDs to handle acuity, agitation, and violence. Finally, as a sizeable benefit in an era of contracting beds, many PES units allow patients to remain in the department for up to 24 hours for treatment and stabilization, reducing risk in a short period of time and obviating the need for hospitalization.

If you are worried about someone who may be at risk of suicide, consult the pages that follow and locate the EDs nearest to you. I have also created an interactive map of all the EDs in the Bay Area. You can access it on the Suicide Risk Resources page of my website at www.merrittmentalhealth.com/suicide-risk. If you have questions, call the ED or its general hospital number and ask them. You will find the phone numbers you need in this chapter as well as on the interactive map.

SAN FRANCISCO

Chinese Hospital (415) 677-2300
845 Jackson Street, San Francisco, CA 94133
www.chinesehospital-sf.org
Main (415) 982-2400

CMPC Saint Luke's Campus (415) 641-6625
3555 Cesar Chavez Street, San Francisco, CA 94110
www.cpmc.org
Main (415) 600-6000

CMPC Davies Campus (415) 600-0600
45 Castro Street, San Francisco, CA 94114
www.cpmc.org
Main (415) 600-6000

CMPC Pacific Campus (415) 600-3333
2333 Buchanan Street, San Francisco, CA 94115
www.cpmc.org
Main (415) 600-6000

CPMC Pediatric (415) 600-4444
3700 California Street, San Francisco, CA 94118
www.cpmc.org
Main (415) 600-6000

Kaiser Permanente San Francisco (415) 833-3300
4131 Geary Avenue, San Francisco, CA 94118
www.kp.org
Main (415) 833-2000

Saint Francis Hospital (415) 353-6300
1150 Bush Street, San Francisco, CA 94109
www.saintfrancismemorial.org
Main (415) 353-6000

Family & Friends
Preparing to Talk About It

In the Introduction to this book, I recommend to family and friends that you directly *Talk About It* with anyone you are concerned may be at risk of suicide. I offer the advice that you should, when ready, take out time for contemplation and process how you would feel if the person died by suicide. I recommend the thoughtful preparation of a loving message that you share with the person at risk and, after delivering it, that you listen. No matter what is said, listen well. Keep three principles at the forefront of your thoughts: Listen. Empathize. Validate.

If you have decided to take this step, you are about to do a powerful thing. When you are ready, look back at the Introduction under the section head "Family and Friends" for more detailed suggestions on what to do, what to say, and how to practice attentive and loving listening during the entirety of your conversation.

Let me suggest that another way to convey your feelings and open dialogue and connection with the person you are concerned about is to write a letter and read it aloud. After you prepare a draft, review and revise it carefully until you get it right. Give it to a trusted other in your life—family member, friend, or therapist—and ask that he or she help you prune away any traces of anger, blame, judgment, correction, or control so the only thing remaining on the page is a message of love. Once you have achieved this, read the letter to the person, hopefully with tears in your eyes. Then listen.

Also, at the right moment, ask if the person is safe. Ask him or her to promise not to take away from you one of the things in the world you care about and love the most—the person you are talking to.

There is more you can do to prepare to *Talk About It*. First, be ready with appropriate referrals and a safety plan. Know where the nearest emergency department is. Know the phone number of your local mobile crisis service, and call them in advance to ask questions and learn how they operate and what their hours are. Understand that if at any time you fear imminent harm to self, 911 is the best resource for obtaining help immediately.

Also, if the person does not already have a therapist or psychiatrist, do research in advance and have on hand referrals to mental health professionals available immediately. Emphasize the importance of seeing a professional. Emphasize the value of both medications and psychotherapy as evidence-based treatments that work synergistically to improve mental health and restore hope.

Saint Mary's Medical Center (415) 750-5700
450 Stanyan Street, San Francisco, CA 94117
www.stmarysmedicalcenter.org
Main (415) 668-1000

San Francisco General Hospital PES (415) 206-8125
1001 Potrero Avenue, San Francisco, CA 94110
www.sfghf.org
Main (415) 206-8000

UCSF Parnassus Hospital (415) 353-1037
505 Parnassus Avenue, San Francisco, CA 94143
www.ucsfhealth.org
Main (415) 476-1000

VA Medical Center San Francisco (415) 221-4810
4150 Clement Street, San Francisco, CA 94121
www.sanfrancisco.va.gov
Main (415) 221-4810

EAST BAY

Alameda Hospital (510) 522-3700
2070 Clinton Avenue, Alameda, CA 94501
www.alamedaahs.org
Main (510) 523-4357

Contra Costa Regional Medical Center PES (925) 646-2800
2500 Alhambra Avenue, Martinez, CA 94553
www.cchealth.org
Main (925) 370-5000

Doctors Medical Center San Pablo Campus (510) 970-5430
2000 Vale Road, San Pablo, CA 94806
www.doctorsmedicalcenter.org
Main (510) 970-5000

Safety Assessment Questions

- When is the last time you had thoughts of harming or killing yourself?
- Are you concerned that you might kill yourself? If so, under what circumstances? What could happen in your life that might prompt serious thoughts of suicide?
- Is anyone close to you concerned that you might commit suicide?
- If you killed yourself, how would you do it?
- When did you last have a thought of any kind about killing yourself? Tell me about it, in detail.
- Are your suicidal thoughts/urges fleeting, frequent, or continual?
- What is the closest you have ever come to committing suicide?
- What are 2-3 reasons for dying? What are 2-3 reasons for living?
- Do you have the means to end your life? Do you have access to weapons or drugs?
- What do you think might make you feel more hopeful?
- Do you think that if you get into a crisis where you feel intensely suicidal that you can call me (or another person/hotline/mobile crisis or go to the emergency department) instead of acting on the impulse?
- What would the impact of your death by suicide be on your family and friends?

Highland Hospital (510) 437-4559
1441 E. 31st Street, Oakland, CA 94602
www.highlandahs.org
Main (510) 437-4800

John George Psychiatric Hospital PES (510) 346-1421
2060 Fairmount Drive, San Leandro, CA 94578
www.johngeorgeahs.org
Main (510) 346-1300

Assessing Hopelessness

- Do you think things will get better?
- Can you name one change that would help turn things around?

John Muir Medical Center Concord (925) 674-3100

2540 East Street, Concord, CA 94520
www.johnmuirhealth.com
Main (925) 682-8200

John Muir Medical Center Walnut Creek (925) 939-5800

1601 Ygnacio Valley Road, Walnut Creek, CA 94598
www.johnmuirhealth.com
Main (925) 939-3000

Kaiser Permanente Antioch (925) 813-6880

4501 Sand Creek Road, Antioch, CA 94531
www.kp.org
Main (925) 813-6500

Kaiser Permanente Fremont (510) 248-7206

39400 Paseo Padre Parkway, Fremont, CA 94538
www.kp.org
Main (510) 248-3000

Kaiser Permanente Oakland (510) 752-7667

3779 Piedmont Avenue, Oakland, CA 94611
www.kp.org
Main (510) 752-1000

Kaiser Permanente Richmond (510) 307-1566

901 Nevin Avenue, Richmond, CA 94804
www.kp.org
Main (510) 307-1500

Kaiser Permanente San Leandro (510) 454-4348
2500 Merced Street, San Leandro, CA 94577
www.kp.org
Main (510) 454-1000

Kaiser Permanente Walnut Creek (925) 295-5100
1425 South Main Street, Walnut Creek, CA 94596
www.kp.org
Main (925) 295-4070

Saint Rose Hospital (510) 264-4026
27200 Calaroga Avenue, Hayward, CA 94545
www. strosehospital.org
Main (510) 264-4000

San Leandro Hospital (510) 357-4545
13855 E 14th Street, San Leandro, CA 94578
www. sanleandroahs.org
Main (510) 667-6500

San Ramon Regional Medical Center (925) 275-8280
6001 Norris Canyon Road, San Ramon, CA 94583
www.sanramonmedctr.com
Main (925) 275-9200

Sutter Alta Bates Summit Medical Center
Alta Bates Campus (510) 204-2500
2450 Ashby Street, Berkeley, CA 94705
www.altabatessummit.org
Main (510) 204-4444

Assessing Methods

- If you committed suicide, how would you do it?
- What methods have you thought about using to commit suicide?
- Do you have the means to commit suicide available now (firearms, pills, chemicals)?

Sutter Alta Bates Summit Medical Center
Summit Campus (510) 869-8700
350 Hawthorne Avenue, Oakland, CA 94609
www.altabatessummit.org
Main (510) 655-4000

Sutter Eden Medical Center (510) 727-3015
13855 East 14th Street, San Leandro, CA 94578
www.altabatessummit.org
Main (510) 727-2703

UCSF Benioff Children's Hospital (510) 428-3240
747 52nd Avenue, Oakland, CA 94601
www.childrenshospitaloakland.org
Main (510) 428-3000

ValleyCare Medical Center (925) 416-3418
5555 West Las Positas Boulevard, Pleasanton, CA 94588
www.valleycare.com
Main (925) 373-4023

Warning Signs of Suicide Risk

- Preoccupation with death
- Statements that life is not worth living
- Direct expression of suicidal thoughts or feelings
- Hopelessness about one's life or future
- Talking about feeling trapped or being in unbearable pain
- Talking about being a burden to others
- Seeming to say goodbye
- Giving away possessions or otherwise making preparations
- Increased use of alcohol or drugs
- Increased anxiety or agitation
- Isolation and withdrawal

Washington Hospital (510) 791-3430
2000 Mowry Avenue, Fremont, CA 94538
www.whhs.com
Main (510) 797-1111

NORTH BAY

Healdsburg District Hospital (707) 431-6300
1375 University Street, Healdsburg, CA 95448
www.healsburgdistricthospital.org
Main (707) 431-6500

Kaiser Permanente San Rafael (415) 444-2400
99 Montecillo Road, San Rafael, CA 94903
www.kp.org
Main (415) 444-2000

Kaiser Permanente Vacaville (707) 624-1160
1 Quality Drive, Vacaville, CA 95688
www.kp.org
Main (707) 624-4000

Kaiser Permanente Vallejo (707) 651-4910
975 Sereno Drive, Vallejo, CA 94590
www.kp.org
Main (707) 651-1000

Marin General Hospital PES (415) 499-6666
250 Bon Air Road, Greenbrae, CA 94904
www.maringeneral.org
Main (415) 925-7000

North Bay Medical Center (707) 646-5800
1200 B Gale Wilson Boulevard, Fairfield, CA 94533
www.northbay.org
Main (707) 646-5000

North Bay Vacavalley Hospital (707) 624-7800
1000 Nut Tree Road, Vacaville, CA 95687
www.northbay.org
Main (707) 624-7000

Novato Community Hospital (415) 209-1350
180 Rowland Way, Novato, CA 94995
www.novatocommunity.org
Main (415) 209-1300

Petaluma Valley Hospital (707) 778-2634
400 North McDowell Boulevard, Petaluma, CA 94954.
www.stjoesonoma.org
Main (707) 778-1111

Queen of the Valley Medical Center (707) 257-4014
1000 Trancas Street, Napa, CA 94558.
www.thequeen.org
Main (707) 252-4411

Saint Helena Hospital (707) 963-6425
10 Woodland Road, Saint Helena, CA 94574
www.adventistihealth.org
Main (707) 963-3611

Santa Rosa Memorial Hospital (707) 525-5207
1165 Montgomery Drive, Santa Rosa, CA 95405
www.stjoesonoma.org
Main (707) 546-3210

Sonoma Valley Hospital (707) 935-5105
347 Andrieux Street, Sonoma, CA 95476
www.svh.com
Main (707) 935-5000

Golden Gate Bridge Safety Project

You may not know that the bridge, perhaps the most beautiful in the world, is also a deadly one. It has more than one legacy. One is of stunning grandeur and elegance, tall ruby orange towers gleaming by day, at night illuminated by a thousand lights, conjuring inspiration and hope. Up close, walking the 1.7 miles between San Francisco and Marin, gusting winds and salt air enhance the magnificent views of ocean, bay, beach, city, and the headlands.

The other legacy is darker: two or three leaps to death every month. They are easy jumps, too, because the railing on the Golden Gate Bridge is unique in its short height--only four feet, one of the lowest of any suspension bridge in the world. The beauty, the grandeur, and this singular physical feature of the bridge afford it another notable: It is the most popular suicide destination site on earth. Other reasons for the bridge's attraction are that death there is not messy and virtually assured.

Since its opening in 1937, thousands have lost their lives. There have been more nearly 1600 official suicides from the bridge, but countless others are undocumented. Three-fourths are male. Ten percent are adolescents. The youngest known to die is a fourteen year old girl, Marissa Imrie, who took a cab fifty miles from her Santa Rosa home to jump. Many more--family, friends, schools, and other communities--are affected by these deaths. Suicide ripples. It is estimated that one suicide directly and intimately affects at least six other people.

The first hard push for a suicide deterrent came in 1948, and still today it remains to be built. John Bateson, author of *The Final Leap: Suicide on the Golden Gate Bridge*, explains why. He says that the twin much-promoted arguments against a barrier--$50 million price tag and aesthetic disfigurement--are surface issues. In an incisive analysis, he insists instead that societal apathy and intransigence stem from shame, stigma, and a faulty belief that bridge deaths would have occurred by other methods of suicide *anyway*. Research reveals this not to be true. Very often a person becomes fixated on a single method of suicide, and if the means is removed the individual survives.

Continued

As far as means go, the bridge is lethal, as lethal as a gunshot to the head. After jumping, a child, young adult, mother, father, brother, sister, aunt, uncle, grandparent, or friend travels at approximately 75 mph 220 feet through the air to water which, on impact, is as solid as rock.

There is good news. Due to the tireless advocacy of some, prominently the Bridge Rail Foundation and the Northern California Psychiatric Foundation, the Bridge authority approved a safety net in October of 2008. The environmental review for the net was completed in February of 2010, and in the spring of 2012 Senator Barbara Boxer authored legislation for funding that passed both houses. In July of that year President Obama signed the bill into law.

According to David Hull, founding president of the Bridge Rail Foundation, the project is at last advancing with true expectancy of success. Final funding was approved by the bridge board in the summer of 2014. A final design received the seal of approval in December. If the current schedule holds, construction of the lifesaving suicide net should be complete in 2018.

Hopefully, after 2018, the dual legacy of the Golden Gate Bridge will slowly be erased. Hopefully the bridge will stand thereafter as the marvelous international monument it deserves to be, freed from easy access over the rail to death in the waters below.

John Bateson, *The Final Leap: Suicide on the Golden Gate Bridge*
(University of California Press, 2012)

Sutter Solano Medical Center (707) 554-5210
300 Hospital Drive, Vallejo, CA 94590
www.suttersolano.org
Main (707) 554-4444

PENINSULA

El Camino Hospital Mountain View (650) 940-7055
2500 Grant Road, Mountain View, CA 94040
www.elcaminohospital.org
Main (650) 940-7000

Kaiser Permanente Redwood City (650) 299-2200
1100 Veterans Boulevard, Redwood City, CA 94603
www.kp.org
Main (650) 299-2000

Kaiser Permanente South San Francisco (650) 742-2511
1200 El Camino Real, South San Francisco, CA 94080
www.kp.org
Main (650) 742-2000

Mills-Peninsula Medical Center PES (650) 696-5915
1501 Trousdale Drive, Burlingame, CA 94010
www.mills-peninsula.org
Main (650) 696-5400

San Mateo Medical Center PES (650) 573-2662
222 West 39th Avenue, San Mateo, CA 94403
www.sanmateomedicalcenter.org
Main (650) 573-2222

Sequoia Hospital (650) 367-5542
170 Alameda de las Pulgas, Redwood City, CA 94062
www.sequoiahospital.org
Main (650) 369-5811

Seton Medical Center (650) 991-6456
1900 Sullivan Avenue, Daly City, CA 94015
www.seton.dochs.org
Main (650) 992-4000

Map of All Bay Area Emergency Departments

I have created an interactive map of all EDs in the Bay Area. You can access it on the Suicide Risk Resources page of my websiite at www.merrittmentalhealth.com/suicide-risk.

Seton Medical Center Coastside (650) 563-7107
600 Marine Boulevard, Moss Beach, CA 94038
www.setoncoastside.org
Main (650) 563-7100

Stanford Hospital (650) 723-5111
300 Pasteur Drive, Palo Alto, CA 94305
www.stanfordhealthcare.org
Main (650) 723-4000

SOUTH BAY

El Camino Hospital Los Gatos (408) 866-4040
815 Pollard Road, Los Gatos, CA 95032
www.elcaminohospital.org
Main (408) 378-6131

Good Samaritan Hospital (408) 559-2552
2425 Samaritan Drive, San Jose, CA 95124
www.goodsamsanjose.com
Main (408) 559-2011

Kaiser Permanente San Jose (408) 972-6140
250 Hospital Parkway, San Jose, CA 95119
www.kp.org
Main (408) 972-3000

Kaiser Permanente Santa Clara (408) 851-5300
700 Lawrence Expressway, Santa Clara, CA 95051
www.kp.org
Main (408) 851-1000

O'Connor Hospital (408) 947-3999
2015 Forest Avenue, San Jose, CA 95128
www.oconnor.dochs.org
Main (408) 947-2500

National Suicide Statistics

- Every day, approximately 105 Americans die by suicide.
- There is one death by suicide in the US every 13 minutes.
- An estimated quarter million people each year become suicide survivors.
- There is one suicide for every estimated 25 suicide attempts.
- Females are more likely than males to have had suicidal thoughts.
- Females attempt suicide three times as often as males (but men die in higher numbers due to effectiveness of methods employed).
- The prevalence of suicidal thoughts, suicidal planning, and suicide attempts is significantly higher among adults aged 18-29 than among adults aged 30+.
- Suicide is the 2nd leading cause of death for 15 to 24-year-old Americans.
- Suicide is the 4th leading cause of death for adults ages 18-65.

Suicide Awareness Voices of Education (SAVE), 2014

Regional Medical Center of San Jose (408) 259-5000 Ext. 2267
225 North Jackson Avenue, San Jose, CA 95116
www.regionalmedicalsanjose.com
Main (408) 259-5000

Saint Louise Regional Hospital (408) 848-2000
9400 North Name Uno, Gilroy, CA 95020
www.saintlouise.dochs.org
Main (408) 848-2000

Santa Clara Valley Medical Center PES (408) 885-6100
751 South Bascom Avenue, San Jose, CA 95128
www.scvmc.org
Main (408) 885-5000

6

Hospital Inpatient Units

In contemporary psychiatric care, emergency departments are the most common and important conduits for inpatient hospitalizations for suicide risk. Patients come to the emergency department, where they are evaluated and sometimes immediately treated for acute conditions like anxiety and agitation. Clinicians conduct a suicide risk assessment and make the determination either to hospitalize or to discharge back home. Typically, if the decision is made to hospitalize, the clinician places the patient on an involuntary 72-hour "hold." If the hospital affiliated with the emergency department has an inpatient unit appropriate for the patient, with an insurance match and beds available, the patient can be admitted there. If not, the patient is typically transported by ambulance to the nearest appropriate inpatient unit at another hospital.

Hospitalization has grown increasingly complex over the past two decades as care has become more expensive and the insurance industry has constricted services. To connect the pieces of the puzzle, please read the introduction to Chapter 4, "Emergency Departments," and the spotlight, "Involuntary 72-Hour Hospitalization," as complements to this chapter. Putting them together will paint a broad picture of acute psychiatric services in the Bay Area and showcase the intricate connections between emergency departments, insurance reimbursement, involuntary legal holds, inpatient units, and the clinicians struggling to make successful linkages between them.

What is the purpose of a psychiatric hospitalization and what happens during a patient's stay? Most experts agree that the twin purposes of hospitalization today are safety and stabilization. A patient is admitted to the hospital not because he or she is depressed, manic, psychotic, or disoriented, but because these mental states engender an imminent danger of harm to self and others. Most psychiatric inpatient units are "locked," meaning that patients cannot come and go freely but instead must have permission or accompaniment to leave the floor. Most have at least one "safe room," a place where a person who is acutely agitated or self-destructive is made safe from potential self-harm from behaviors like head banging or self-hitting with hard objects. Safe rooms, however, are for emergencies only. They are not for typical inpatient hospitalization. Most patients rest comfortably in a standard hospital room.

Safety is the first aim of a psychiatric hospitalization. Stabilization is the process of calming the acute internal emotional state that spurred the admission. Numerous aspects of care offered in inpatient units help to accomplish this. One is removal of the individual from the acute stressors of the outside world: living situations, relationship conflicts, and the pressure of work or academics. Another source of relief is medications, whether the prescription of a new treatment regimen or adjustments to a current one. Hospitals also provide stabilization through individual psychotherapy, group therapy, and education about mental illness and coping. Finally, relief can come from family sessions, wherein family members come to better understand the condition at hand and how to respond most effectively to the suffering of their loved ones. Family sessions are also opportunities for patients and family members to speak openly, to listen, and to repair damage in their relationships.

Beyond safety and stabilization, there is a third vital goal of psychiatric hospitalization that is often underappreciated: the aftercare plan. That is, what is the outpatient discharge plan for ensuring safety, stability, and ongoing treatment and clinical improvement in the outside world? Who is the therapist? Who is the physician? Have appointments been set up in advance to assure continuity of care? What about groups, social support, family therapy, IOPs, PHPs, residential treatment centers, and addiction treatment? Have these been considered and set in place *prior to discharge*?

Over and over in my consultations with patients and families, I emphasize that *the single most important objective* of a psychiatric hospitalization is a comprehensive aftercare plan. Safety and stabilization happened automatically. This is hardly true of good aftercare. Hospital staff are busy. Social workers organizing discharge are confronted by the same challenges everyone else faces in contemporary mental health care: disarray, fragmentation, and insurance company resistance to cover recommended care. Discharge planners do their best, but their time is limited. Sometimes a patient may be discharged with a simple recommendation to find a psychiatrist or a list of several names of therapists or psychiatrists but no firm appointments yet established.

This is insufficient. I cannot repeat often enough: Nothing is more important upon discharge than a *comprehensive aftercare plan*. Patients and family members must advocate for themselves on this essential component of care. They must insist that discharge positively not occur until a solid aftercare plan has been agreed upon.

Planning should begin the same day of admission. Ask staff to refer you to the social worker who will be in charge of discharge. Set up an appointment, and speak with that person. Say you understand that aftercare is sometimes a weak link in the hospital process and that you are invested in setting up an excellent plan and want to go to work immediately in collaboration with staff to achieve that end.

Family members should never wonder what they can do during the course of a hospitalization to be helpful. They should participate fully in family meetings, listen, and learn as much as possible. They should take the opportunity to develop listening skills and the art of soft, loving responses. They should become unrelenting aftercare advocates. They should invest whatever time necessary on the phone, on the Internet, and in consultation with mental health experts to develop an excellent aftercare plan. To repeat, no component of inpatient hospital care is more important than the aftercare plan.

SAN FRANCISCO

CMPC Pacific Campus (415) 600-3252
2333 Buchanan Street, San Francisco, CA 94115
www.cpmc.org
Main (415) 600-6000

Saint Francis Hospital (415) 353-6230
1150 Bush Street, San Francisco, CA 94109
www.saintfrancismemorial.org
Main (415) 353-6000

Saint Mary's Medical Center (415) 750-5649
450 Stanyan Street, San Francisco, CA 94117
www.stmarysmedicalcenter.org
Main (415) 668-1000

San Francisco General Hospital (415) 206-6300
1001 Potrero Avenue, San Francisco, CA 94110
www.sfghf.org
Main (415) 206-8000

VA Medical Center San Francisco (415) 221-2073
4150 Clement Street, San Francisco, CA 94121
www.sanfrancisco.va.gov
Main (415) 221-4810

EAST BAY

Contra Costa Regional Medical Center (925) 370-5389
2500 Alhambra Avenue, Martinez, CA 94553
www.cchealth.org
Main (925) 370-5000

Fremont Hospital Adolescent & Adult Units (510) 796-1100
39001 Sundale Drive, Fremont, CA 94538
www.fremonthospital.com
Main (510) 796-1100

John George Psychiatric Hospital (510) 346-1411
2060 Fairmount Drive, San Leandro, CA 94578
www.johngeorgeahs.org
Main (510) 346-1300

John Muir Medical Center Concord (925) 674-4100
2540 East Street, Concord, CA 94520
www.johnmuirhealth.com
Main (925) 682-8200

NORTH BAY

Aurora Hospital (414) 454-6777, Ext. 1
1287 Fulton Road, Santa Rosa, CA 94501
www.aurorasantarosa.com
Main (414) 454-6777

Marin General Hospital (415) 925-7663
250 Bon Air Road, Greenbrae, CA 94904
www.maringeneral.org
Main (415) 925-7000

Saint Helena Hospital (707) 963-6270
10 Woodland Road, Saint Helena, CA 94574
www.adventistihealth.org
Main (707) 963-3611

PENINSULA

El Camino Hospital Mountain View (650) 940-7291
2500 Grant Road, Mountain View, CA 94040
www.elcaminohospital.org
Main (650) 940-7000

Guardedness?
An Essential Question to Reduce Resistance

I have found over the years that patients are greatly interested in talking about suicidal thoughts and feelings in clinical interviews and sessions with me. However, not infrequently I detect an emergent discomfort with my questions related to suicide risk. There may be fidgeting, guardedness, short answers, and an appearance of minimizing. When this happens, I pause and say:

> "Let me ask you. Are you concerned that how you answer these questions might lead me to hospitalize you against your will?"

These can be powerful words. Many patients experience this fear and are relieved to have it brought out into the open. Often this singular question—and the dialogue that follows—quickly shifts the feeling in the room from one of guarded anxiety to calm and trust.

After listening well, I let patients know that hospitalization is a last resort I never turn to lightly. I explain that the purpose of hospitalization is to save the life of a person at imminent risk of death when no other plan seems safe. It is not a first-line course of action for suicidal thoughts, feelings, or plans without imminent risk.

Invariably, this simple intervention in my office dissipates anxiety and guardedness, allowing the assessment to proceed in an honest, self-revelatory direction.

Mills-Peninsula Medical Center
Adolescent (650) 696-4600 **& Adult** (650) 696-4650
1501 Trousdale Drive, Burlingame, CA 94010
www.mills-peninsula.org
Main (650) 696-5400

San Mateo Medical Center (650) 573-2760
222 West 39th Avenue, San Mateo, CA 94403
www.sanmateomedicalcenter.org
Main (650) 573-2222

Essential Checklist for Suicide Risk Assessment

- ☐ Assessed for current active mood, anxiety, psychotic, and substance use disorders
- ☐ Assessed for hopelessness/despairing view of future
- ☐ Assessed for wish to be dead
- ☐ Assessed for current suicidal ideation, plan, intent, and imminence
- ☐ Assessed for access to means
- ☐ Assessed for guardedness vs. reliability in responses given
- ☐ Obtained history of past suicidal ideation and attempts
- ☐ Considered risk factors and protective factors
- ☐ A Crisis Plan was established and credibly agreed upon
- ☐ Patient reassessed at end of clinical interview
- ☐ In the case of high risk in a guarded patient, collateral history was obtained from family members/friends
- ☐ In the case of imminent danger to self, a safety plan/hospitalization protocol was followed
- ☐ Where there is risk but no imminent danger to self, an appropriate treatment and follow-up plan was established

Stanford Hospital (650) 723-5868
300 Pasteur Drive, Palo Alto, CA 94305
www.stanfordhealthcare.org
Main (650) 723-4000

SOUTH BAY

Good Samaritan Hospital (408) 358-5652
2425 Samaritan Drive, San Jose, CA 95124
www.goodsamsanjose.com
Main (408) 559-2011

Kaiser Permanente Santa Clara (408) 851-4850
700 Lawrence Expressway, Santa Clara, CA 95051
www.kp.org
Main (408) 851-1000

Santa Clara Valley Medical Center (408) 885-6220
751 South Bascom Avenue, San Jose, CA 95128
www.scvmc.org
Main (408) 885-5000

7

Crisis Stabilization Units

This chapter outlines resources on an intermediate level between emergency department care and inpatient psychiatric care: crisis stabilization units. These services are expanding nationally and hold great promise of helping doctors, patients, and family members steer clear of unnecessary and sometimes unproductive visits to the emergency department as well as unnecessary hospitalizations.

Crisis stabilizations units are specialized short-term psychiatric emergency services designed to provide the full scope of assessment, management, referrals, and case management to patients who present in distress. What makes them different and often superior to emergency department care is their expertise in psychiatric disorders. Crisis units are staffed not by general medicine emergency department staff, but by mental health professionals. They are trained in sensitive interview techniques and comprehensive risk assessment. They are more knowledgeable about local outpatient psychiatric services and make referrals that more aptly fit a patient's specific needs. Added to this, some units have short-term beds where patients can "stabilize." In this regard, they are a valuable alternative to hospitalization.

To further understand crisis stabilization services and the vital current and future role they have to play in acute psychiatric care, it is helpful to briefly review the process of assessing and managing suicide risk in contemporary psychiatric care.

In this process, a clinician begins with screening questions about suicidal thoughts and feelings. For example, "Have you recently been having thoughts that life is not worth living or that you would rather be dead?" More specific to active suicidal risk, "How about thoughts of taking your own life?" The clinician listens empathically, conveying an attitude of calm and open acceptance of the patient's suicidal thoughts and feelings.

Acknowledgement of thoughts of suicide—what doctors call *suicidal ideation*—spurs the next phase of evaluation: a full suicide risk assessment. Here the clinician explores in greater detail the following components of risk, among others: 1) the content of suicidal thoughts 2) risk factors 3) methods contemplated 4) presence or absence of a current or past plan for suicide 5) strength of desire for death 6) intent to follow a plan and 7) imminence of intent.

Typically, in both the Bay Area and nationally, the finding of a present plan with *imminent* intent to die by suicide triggers an involuntary hospitalization. In past decades hospitalization was not a hurried experience exclusively focused on safety and short-term stabilization. There was less time pressure. Patients sometimes stayed for a week or two, adjusting medications and attending educational lectures, group therapies, and family therapy sessions. Today, to the minds of many experts, hospitalization has become little more than a costly inpatient stabilization service. The purpose is rapid stabilization followed by rapid discharge to outpatient care.

Specialized outpatient crisis stabilization units are now offering the same service at less expense in a single location. There is no need for conducting difficult searches for scarce hospital beds. There is no need for expensive transport services to inpatient units across the city or across the Golden Gate Bridge or Bay Bridge. Stabilization units, generally publicly financed for the uninsured, are designed to aid patients and families through the entire cycle of care, beginning with screening and assessment and extending from there to treatment planning, care coordination, and referrals, all provided under a single roof.

Perhaps no aspect of psychiatric care deserves greater study and expansion than crisis stabilization units. As noted, the vast majority of these facilities in the United States are county services, not available to private insurance patients. The private sector should scrutinize them well and learn from the excellent comprehensive care crisis stabilization units often provide.

SAN FRANCISCO

Dore Urgent Care Center (415) 553-3100
52 Dore Street. San Francisco, CA 94103. www.progressfounda-tion.org. 24/7. A crisis stabilization service in San Francisco avail-able to adults experiencing escalating emotional crisis. Provides assessment and triage in a supportive, community-based setting as an alternative to hospitalization. Refers clients to the Dore House residential program if deemed appropriate. Dore Urgent Care Cen-ter stresses that patients call before coming in.

Edgewood Center for Children and Families (415) 969-4135
1801 Vicente Street, San Francisco, CA 94116. www.edgewood.org. An organization providing crisis stabilization services, hospital di-version services, intensive mental health support in the IOP and PHP levels, and school-based programming.

EAST BAY

Family, Youth and Children's Services
of Berkeley and Albany (510) 981-5280
3282 Adeline Street, Berkeley, CA 94704. www.ci.berkeley.ca.us. An organization providing intensive crisis stabilization and mental health support services to youth and adolescents. Also offers psy-chological assessment and outpatient counseling services, includ-ing individual, family, and brief treatment.

Telecare's Contra Costa Hope House (925) 313-7980
300 Ilene Street, Martinez, CA   94553. www.telecarecorp.com. 24/7. A short-term crisis stabilization residential facility meant as a step-down program or alternative to inpatient hospitalization. The average stay for residents is two weeks.

Officer Kevin Briggs
Guardian of the Golden Gate

On a bright January morning I interviewed Office Kevin Briggs of the California Highway Patrol. I reached out to him for the purpose of learning about his sensitive manner and technique of engaging with individuals on the Golden Gate Bridge at risk of jumping.

Now retired after more than two decades in law enforcement and pursuing a second career in suicide prevention, Officer Briggs intervened with over 200 individuals standing on the precipice of life and death on the bridge. Of these, he lost two. All the rest came back over the rail to safety and a second chance at life.

Before our conversation, I knew I was going to encounter an effective, patient professional. What surprised me about Briggs was something more profound: his deep empathy and big heart. More than anything, I was struck by this remarkable quality in a burly, physically imposing man trained to be tough and hard fighting.

What he related to me about his experiences saving lives on the Golden Gate Bridge reinforced within me a core belief—that is, meeting a person in suicidal crisis with a loving, open heart is the *first principle* of intervention, management, and prevention.

When Briggs approaches a suicidal person on the bridge, he first keeps a respectful distance, asking permission to come closer. His desire is that the person over the rail will not jump. His personal agenda, however, is something different: to listen, to understand, to serve as a touchstone for the restoration of hope.

Today he dedicates much of his time to training law enforcement officials, and in our talk he named "ego" as the greatest obstacle to intervening successfully in acute crisis. He did not mean the ego of the suicidal person, but of the helper.

"You can't control," he emphasized, "You can't order the person like a drill sergeant. You have to stop, fall silent, and listen, listen, listen." The two words he repeated most often during our interview were "listen" and "empathy."

Sometimes bracing against bone-chilling winds and fog deep into the night, once for eight uninterrupted hours, Briggs enters into a warm, caring conversation. Listening attentively, sometimes sharing stories of personal close encounters with death, he perse-

Continued

veres until the person requests his help in coming back over the rail.

What ignites the emotional shift back to life? I think it is Briggs' humility and empathy tied to something else extraordinary: his personal commitment to the life of the person he is speaking with. No one on the bridge feels Officer Briggs is simply doing his job. They know—deep down—that Briggs wants them to live and believes they can live. His commitment and compassion are transforming.

One man who came back over the rail, after hours in conversation with Briggs, was asked afterwards why he changed his mind. What made the difference?

"Kevin would not give up," he said.

Empathy. Humility. Caring. Sincerity. Solace. Perseverance. Commitment. Listening.

These are some of the component parts of Officer Briggs' "technique" for helping those in suicidal crisis. The foundation stone holding them all in place is compassionate listening.

"Listen, listen, listen," he said.

You can read more about Officer Briggs and his suicide prevention methods in his recent book, *Guardian of the Golden Gate: Protecting the Line Between Hope and Despair*. It is essential reading for anyone interested in learning about suicide prevention, generally, and, specifically, in the San Francisco Bay Area.

Telecare's Heritage Psychiatric
Health Facility (510) 535-5115

2633 East 27th Street, Oakland, CA 94601. www.telecarecorp.com. 24 hours, 7 days a week. A short-term locked residential program for people 18 years old and older experiencing a high level of distress symptoms from serious mental health complications. Many of the clients in this facility are at moderate suicide risk and need a higher level of care then an outpatient facility.

Telecare's Sausal Creek
Outpatient Stabilization Clinic (510) 437-2363

2620 26th Avenue, Oakland, CA 94601. www.telecarecorp.com. Monday to Friday: 8:00 a.m. to 8:00 p.m.; Saturday: 8:00 a.m. to

4:30 p.m. A crisis stabilization outpatient clinic available to adults. Psychiatrists refer clients to the best form of longer-term or higher-level care, whether that be a voluntary or involuntary hospitalization in a psychiatric hospital or appropriate outpatient psychiatric services.

Telecare's Willow Rock Center (510) 895-5502

2050 Fairmont Drive, San Leandro, CA 94578. www.telecarecorp. com. A walk-in crisis stabilization unit and an inpatient psychiatric facility for children and adolescents. Clients are referred to Willow Rock either by the police, an emergency department, an outpatient program, or on a self-referral basis. Willow Rock Center offers suicide assessments for all clients as well as detailed care planning for people who do not need inpatient hospitalization. Outpatient services are available at Willow Rock until a more appropriate longer-term facility is located. **Note:** East Bay youth at risk of suicide are most likely to be transferred to Willow Rock from an emergency department. Youth in need of hospitalization should go here first.

NORTH BAY

Children's Crisis Services (707) 253-4711

2344 Old Sonoma Road, Building D, Napa, CA 94559. www.countyofnapa.org. A mental health program providing crisis services

---

Essential Components of Systematic Risk Assessment When Suicidal Ideation is Present

- Assess for past suicidal thinking, feeling, and behavior
- Assess for current plan, preparation, intent, means, and imminence
- Assess for risk factors and protective factors
- Develop a near-term and long-term management plan

Essential Elements of Assessment

- Past history of suicidal thoughts, behaviors, attempts
- Present psychiatric illness
- Present substance use disorder
- Hopelessness
- Other risk & protective factors
- Current thoughts of suicide
- Suicide plan
- Suicidal intent
- Imminence of intent

to children and adolescents. Offers assessment, intervention, and stabilization services to children at suicide risk or serious mental distress.

Fairfield Crisis Stabilization Unit (707) 428-1131

675 Texas Street, Suite 4700, Fairfield, CA 94533. 24/7. A walk-in intervention service for adolescents and adults in Solano county.

Napa County Psychiatric Emergency Response Unit (707) 253-4711

2344 Old Sonoma Road, Building D, Napa, CA 94559. www.countyofnapa.org. 24/7. A crisis intervention service for people in Napa Country.

Napa County Intensive Outpatient Program (707) 253-4063

2344 Old Sonoma Road, Building D, Napa, CA 94559. www.countyofnapa.org. An IOP that offers a variety of services including crisis stabilization, 1-on-1 counseling, group counseling and support around relapse and drug recovery.

PENINSULA

Edgewood San Carlos (650) 832-6900

957 Industrial Road, Suite B, San Carlos, CA 94070. www.edgewood.com. A treatment center for children and adolescents ages 6 to 14. Provides crisis stabilization and long-term planning to reduce high-risk behaviors.

SOUTH BAY

EMQ Families First Crisis Stabilization Unit (408) 364-4083

251 Llewellyn Avenue, Campbell, CA 95008. www.emqff.org. A 24/7 crisis intervention service for children and adolescents in Santa Clara County.

8

Hospital-Based PHPs & IOPs

One of the most important questions a psychiatrist, psychologist, teacher, or family member must address in deciding on the best treatment pathway for someone with suicide risk centers on "level of care." What level of care will ensure the patient's safety, first, and, second, optimize health outcomes?

My own goal in consulting and providing best referrals is to help patients *to get as well as they can as soon as they can*. This is the chief operating principle on my mind every day with each recommendation and referral I make. The associated salient question is easy to pose: What is the best level of care for this patient at this time? Providing the answer, however, is much more challenging since it requires integrating the doctor's recommendations with patient preferences and various limitations of work, school, timing, location, program availability, insurance reimbursement, and financial wherewithal to pay for services.

Here is one hierarchy of levels of psychiatric care, from highest to lowest:

- Inpatient
- Residential
- Partial Hospitalization Program (PHP)
- Intensive Outpatient Program (IOP)
- Outpatient twice weekly with clinician, plus group
- Outpatient twice weekly
- Outpatient weekly
- Outpatient biweekly, monthly, or less

The first two levels of care involve overnight stays at the hospital or treatment center. The rest are outpatient pathways in which the number of hours spent in treatment varies from 40-50 hours per week in a PHP, at one extreme, to a 15-minute "med check" once every 3-4 months for a patient who is stable and simply needs infrequent monitoring and refills.

This chapter provides a comprehensive list of all hospital-based PHPs (partial hospitalization programs) and IOPs (intensive outpatient programs) in the Bay Area. What are these day programs, and what is the difference between them? I like to think of both types of programs as "schools for emotional healing and learning." They offer comprehensive, short-term intensive treatment. Individuals attend structured programming throughout the day, three to seven days a week, and return home in the evenings. IOPs and PHPs are places people go to speed up the process of healing and recovery, especially when lower levels of care are not successfully achieving safety and stability.

Primarily, the difference between the two is a matter of intensity as reflected in the numbers of days per week or hours per day a patient spends in the program. In fact, every partial hospitalization program is an intensive outpatient program. A better way to differentiate them would be to rename them "IOP Level I" (IOP) and "IOP Level II" (PHP). IOPs typically run 8-15 hours per week and PHPs 30-40 hours. That's the main difference.

What do the programs offer? The offerings break down into five dominant categories: medication treatment, individual therapy, group therapy, family therapy, and mental health education ("psychoeducation," it is often called). Here is an expanded list of typical components of treatment and education:

- Assessment & diagnosis
- Treatment planning
- Individual therapy
- Family therapy
- Cognitive Behavior Therapy groups
- Dialectical Behavior Therapy groups
- Relationship-focused therapy groups
- Medication management
- Interpersonal skills training
- Occupational therapy
- Social skills training
- Stress reduction
- Yoga-relaxation training
- Mindfulness meditation
- Spiritual counseling
- Education groups
- Life planning and goal setting
- Aftercare planning

What I like most about PHPs and IOPs is that they are immersive treatments. We all know that the only truly successful way to learn a language is through "immersion." I believe the same is true of emotional growth and recovery from mental illness and/or addiction.

Find excellent treatment and get immersed in it—for as many hours per day as possible. This is the most promising pathway for getting as well as you can as soon as you can.

IOPs and PHPs vary widely in the populations served and services provided, so make sure to research them well as you consider which one offers the best fit for you, your family member, or your patient. If you are looking for specialty programs—adolescent, geriatric, substance abuse, eating disorder, or other diagnoses—simply ask the admissions director of any program for further advice, direction, and guidance.

SAN FRANCISCO

UCSF Parnassus Hospital/Langley Porter PHP (415) 476-7832
401 Parnassus Avenue, San Francisco, CA 94143
www.ucsfhealth.org
Main (415) 476-9000

EAST BAY

Alameda Health System at
Highland Hospital PHP & IOP (510) 535-7476
1411 East 31st Street, Oakland, CA 94602
www.highlandahs.org
Main (510) 437-4800

Fremont Hospital PHP & IOP (510) 574-4851
39001 Sundale Drive, Fremont, CA 94538
www.fremonthospital.com
Main (510) 796-110

John Muir Medical Center Concord PHP & IOP (925) 674-4140
2740 Grant Street, Concord, CA 94520
www.johnmuirhealth.com
Main (925) 682-8200

Kaiser Permanente Antioch IOP (925) 777-6300
3454 Hill Crest Avenue, Antioch, CA 94531
www.kp.org
Main (925) 813-6500

Kaiser Permanente Oakland IOP (510) 752-7394
3900 Broadway Boulevard, Oakland, CA 94611
www.kp.org
Main (510) 752-1000

Involuntary 72-Hour Hospitalization

In the Emergency Department at Stanford Hospital as a psychiatric resident during three years of training, I placed dozens of patients on "5150 Involuntary Holds." On each occasion I assessed risk of "danger to self," as a primary concern, and "voluntariness," as secondary.

In those years, 1999-2002, when a suicidal person was willing to be admitted voluntarily, we rarely issued a 5150 (a legal order necessitating a 72-hour detention and observation period in a locked psychiatric ward). With rare exception, all the 5150s I wrote were in cases of patient refusal to be hospitalized, where the risk seemed high enough to legally intervene for the purpose of safety.

Times have changed. Today, at least in many hospitals in Northern California, it has become a standard to issue a 5150 even when the patient is willing to be hospitalized on a voluntary basis.

Why this shift? To discover the answer, I spoke with a half dozen colleagues in emergency psychiatry. They seemed to agree generally on four essential contributing factors.

Compared to a voluntary hospitalization, a 5150 ensures: 1) greater patient safety 2) greater confidence in gaining an actual admission to the hospital 3) enhanced liability protection for peace officers and health professionals in the event of adverse outcomes and 4) higher reimbursement from insurance companies for hospitalizations.

Hence, when a 5150 is included as part of the admission process, a patient tends to be kept safer and to stand a higher chance of securing a bed. Moreover, the patient will more consistently win the argument of "medical necessity"—even *legal necessity*—when insurance representatives attempt to deny coverage.

No doubt, 5150s strip citizens of their civil rights. A 72-hour legal detention is a serious matter never to be embraced lightly. Even so, for people in crisis who are willing to be admitted voluntarily, these legal writs have become routine. In many cases, they offer tangible benefits to patients and family members at times of uncertainty and life-and-death fear.

Medications in the Management of Acute Suicide Risk

- Treat agitation
- Treat anxiety
- Treat depression
- Treat psychosis

Kaiser Permanente Fremont IOP (510) 248-3060

39400 Paseo Padre Parkway, Fremont, CA 94538
www.kp.org
Main (510) 248-3000

Kaiser Permanente Union City IOP (510) 675-3080

3555 Whipple Road, Union City, CA 94587
www.kp.org
Main (510) 675-4010

Kaiser Permanente Richmond IOP (510) 307-1591

901 Nevin Avenue, Richmond, CA 94801
www.kp.org
Main (510) 307-1500

Kaiser Permanente Walnut Creek IOP (925) 295-4145

710 South Main Street, Walnut Creek, CA 94596
www.kp.org
Main (925) 295-4070

Sutter Alta Bates Summit Medical Center
Herrick Campus PHP & IOP (510) 204-4469

2001 Dwight Way, Berkeley, CA 94704
www.altabatessummit.org
Main (510) 204-4460

NORTH BAY

Aurora Hospital PHP & IOP (707) 800-7700
1287 Fulton Road, Santa Rosa, CA 94501
www.aurorasantarosa.com
Main (707) 800-7700

Kaiser Permanente San Rafael IOP (415) 491-3000
111 Smith Ranch Road, San Rafael, CA 94903
www.kp.org
Main (415) 444-2000

Kaiser Permanente Vacaville IOP (707) 624-2830
1 Quality Drive, Vacaville, CA 95688
www.kp.org
Main (707) 624-4000

Kaiser Permanente Vallejo IOP (707) 651-1025
975 Sereno Drive, Vallejo, CA 94590
www.kp.org
Main (707) 651-1000

Marin General Hospital PHP & IOP (415) 925-7633
250 Bon Air Road, Greenbrae, CA 94904
www.maringeneral.org
Main (415) 925-7000 7663

Evidence-Based Biological Interventions

- Lithium & clozapine
- Antidepressants
- Atypical antipsychotics
- Electroconvulsive Therapy and Transcranial Magnetic Stimulation
- Ketamine

Griffiths, *American Journal of Preventive Medicine*,
September 2014

Saint Helena Hospital PHP (707) 649-4925
525 Oregon Street, Saint Helena, CA 94574
www.adventistihealth.org
Main (707) 963-3611

PENINSULA

**El Camino Hospital Mountain View
PHP & IOP** (650) 940-7254
2500 Grant Road, Mountain View, CA 94040
www.elcaminohospital.org
Main (650) 940-7000

Mills Health Center PHP & IOP (650) 696-4690
100 South San Mateo Drive, San Mateo, CA 94401
www.mills-peninsula.org
Main (650) 696-5400

SOUTH BAY

Good Samaritan Hospital IOP (408) 559-2000
2425 Samaritan Drive, San Jose, CA 95124
www.goodsamsanjose.com
Main (408) 559-2011

Kaiser Permanente Santa Clara IOP (408) 366-4400
19000 East Homestead Road, Cupertino, CA 95014
www.kp.org
Main (408) 851-1000

9

Clinics

"Clinics" represent the greatest area of growth in mental health services related to suicide risk. Throughout the Bay Area, gaining access to general psychiatric care is challenging at best. Yet there is a special paradox when it comes to suicide risk. Whenever the words "suicide" or "suicidal thoughts" are expressed in relation to a patient, all voices counsel family members, friends, educators, and patients themselves: "Go to the emergency department."

However, emergency room physicians are hardly the only clinicians capable of conducting a careful suicide risk assessment, and they offer little treatment beyond short-term calming agents. The paradox lies in the fact that emergency departments are hospitalizing fewer and fewer patients with suicide risk, but they are still the only reliable, recommended clinical setting available for same-day assessments. Patients wait long hours in sterile, sometimes noisy and disruptive waiting rooms only to be told after a brief evaluation to return home and find an outpatient doctor for follow-up.

What this means is that the Bay Area stands in drastic need of more easily accessible clinics for evaluation, treatment, referrals, case management, and care navigation. There are insufficient clinics on all shores of the Bay, most notably same-day and next-day walk-in clinics, whether financed by public insurance, private insurance, or private pay. Imagine how this compounds crises of suicide risk for patients, family members, and educators. The first crisis is the suicide risk and the panic and fear it engenders. The second crisis is that of poor, clumsy access to care.

It is not only that Bay Area residents do not know where to turn for urgent evaluation and treatment. To exaggerate the point, there is nowhere to turn. That is, except emergency departments which typically return patients back home with little support and guidance after a lengthy waiting process.

My hope is that in future editions of this book, the resources listed in this chapter will expand exponentially. If you know of clinics or group practices that deserve inclusion, please let us know at info@merrittmentalhealth.com.

Ideally, same-day clinics with expertise in assessing and managing suicide risk will one day be widely available in the Bay Area, with doors open for walk-ins 8 a.m. to 5 p.m. Only when a crisis strikes after normal business hours should a routine evaluation necessarily take place in the emergency department.

SAN FRANCISCO

OMI Family Center (415) 452-2200
1760 Ocean Avenue, San Francisco, CA 94112. www.ymcasf.org. Monday to Friday: 8:30 a.m. to 5:00 p.m. Provides assessment, evaluation, crisis intervention, individual and group counseling, and medication consultations for children and adolescents ages 3 to 18. Clients must be eligible to receive services from Community Behavioral Health Services (CBHS).

Huckleberry Youth Services (415) 751-8181
555 Cole Street, San Francisco, CA 94117. www.huckleberryyouth. org. Monday, Tuesday, Wednesday, Friday: 9:00 a.m. to 5:00 p.m.; Thursday: 2:00 pm to 6:00 pm. Provides assessment on appointment and drop-in basis as well as evaluation and crisis intervention. Serves adolescents and adults ages 11 to 24 living in San Francisco.

Larkin Street Youth Services (415) 673-0911 Ext. 259
1138 Sutter Street, San Francisco, CA. www.larkinstreetyouth.org. Monday, Wednesday, Thursday, Friday: 9:00 a.m. to 5:00 p.m.; Tuesday: 11:00 a.m. to 5:00 p.m. Provides assessment, evaluation, and crisis intervention to homeless youth and adults ages 11 to 24 living in San Francisco.

Merritt Mental Health (415) 285-3774
3786 20th Street, San Francisco, CA 94110. www.merrittmental-health.com. A psychiatric care navigation and health services consultancy. Provides in-person and phone consultations for a fee on any question related to mental health services. Conducts workshops and trainings in suicide risk identification and management.

Mind Therapy Clinic San Francisco
Intensive Outpatient Program (415) 567-4604
2299 Post Street, Suite 104A, San Francisco, CA 94115. Provides assessment, evaluation, medication consultation, individual psychotherapy, group therapy, and substance use support for children, teens, and young adults.

Management of Risk in Solo Practice

Managing suicide risk in solo practice is far more challenging than doing so in a hospital or clinic setting. The primary reason for this is that the clinician has no one immediately available to help and no Emergency Department a short, easy walk away. I have talked to dozens of doctors and therapists in private practice, and there is one critical recurring theme: They positively do not want to call the police and request that an officer come to the practice and then, after a knock on the door, watch their patient be handcuffed and carried off in the back of a police car to a locked ward under a 5150.

Why this reluctance? Because they care about their patients, and this pathway to hospitalization seems uncivilized, unwarranted, and a touch brutal. It is. They are right. Clinicians are also scared of liability. You are not *supposed* to walk with your patient to the Emergency Department, drive your patient in your own car, ride in a cab with your patient—all the civilized, humane things a kind, thinking person would do in the circumstance. What if the patient runs, escapes, or jumps in front of a car on the way? We in the United States worry incessantly about these rare eventualities. We worry about being blamed. We worry about being sued. So, how does our society and its mental health leadership deal with these worries and fears? Handcuffs and police cars.

It is my belief that many mental health professionals avoid admitting patients with suicide risk into their practices for precisely this reason. The "system" is controlling and unforgiving. The system is inhumane. The system will blame you and sue you. These external forces rattle and scare doctors and therapists, so understandably many opt out of clinical work with patients with suicide risk.

There are other reasons that solo clinicians are discomfited by suicide risk. One is that they feel unprepared by lack of good training. Another is that, even when decently trained, they may not see moderate to severe suicide risk in their practices frequently enough to remember what to do. Finally, many doctors and therapists feel deep uncertainty about exactly when the threshold for hospitalization has been reached.

There are a few strategies that can ameliorate these tensions and boost the confidence of solo mental health professionals to work with patients with suicide risk. For one, use your clinical judgment making all decisions. Be informed by rules, regulations, and universal standards, but do not be derailed by them. Clinical judgment is the best compass we have. Use it to the fullest extent possible it to navigate the maze.

Another strategy is to *Talk About It*. If you are in the office with a patient and you feel a lack of confidence, pick up the phone and call a hotline or mobile crisis service. The person who picks up the phone is trained and ready to help.

Tell the patient, "I am concerned about suicide risk. We are going to call a suicide prevention hotline and get a second opinion." Then make the call and turn on the speaker. Be honest and humble. Tell the suicide risk expert you feel unsure and want help. Let him or her do an assessment while you listen, and by the end of the phone call your confidence level will rise. In this wise collaboration a solid plan will form, and you will have offered the best care possible to your patient.

When in doubt, *Talk About It*.

Pacific Coast Psychiatric Associates (415) 296-5290

490 Post Street, Suite 1043, San Francisco, CA 94102. www.pcpasf. com. Hours vary. An association of psychiatrists and psychologists. Provides assessment and treatment for a number of mental health conditions. Explores multiple aspects of patients' lives, including biological, psychological, and social factors to ensure the best treatment.

Southeast Mission Geriatric Services (415) 337-2400

3905 Mission Street, San Francisco, CA. 94112. www.sfdph.org. Monday to Friday: 9:00 a.m. to 5:00 p.m. A service of San Francisco Department of Public Health (SFDPH). Offers crisis stabilization, assessment, case management, and group support in clients' homes and in the community to adults ages 60 and older living in the Southeast district of San Francisco, including the Outer Mission and the Excelsior.

SOMA Mental Health Services (415) 836-1700

760 Harrison Street, San Francisco, CA 94107. www.sfdph.org. Regular hours: Monday, Tuesday, Thursday, Friday: 8:30 a.m. to 5:00 p.m.; Wednesday: 8:30 a.m. to 1:00 p.m. Drop-in hours: Monday to Friday: 8:30 am to 10:00 pm. A service of San Francisco Department of Public Health (SFDPH). Provides assessments, evaluations and medication consultation services to adults ages 18 to 59 living in the SOMA, Tenderloin, and Western Addition neighborhoods. Appointments and drop-in services available.

Stonewall Project (415) 487-3100

1035 Market Street, 4th Floor, San Francisco, CA 94103. A clinic that offers harm reduction counseling to gay men and MSM with substance and mental health conditions. Offers by-appointment counseling and drop-in support Monday to Friday at 4 p.m. Provides services to people currently or previously at risk of suicide.

Suicide Risk Factors

- History of suicide attempts or self-injurious behavior
- Suicidal thoughts, plan, preparation, and/or intent
- Mental health disorder
- Substance use disorder
- Lethal means available
- Isolation
- Recent loss or other painful prompting events
- Hopelessness
- Depression with apathy and loss of interest in life
- Depression with anxiety, panic, and insomnia
- Depression with psychotic thoughts
- Chronic physical pain
- High impulsivity
- Family history of suicide
- Barriers to mental health access

Tom Waddell Urgent Care Clinic (415) 355-7400

230 Golden Gate Avenue, San Francisco, CA 94102. www.twtrans-genderclinic.org. Monday to Friday: 8:00 a.m. to 4:00 p.m.; Saturday: 8:30 a.m. to 3:00 p.m. A service of San Francisco Department of Public Health (SFDPH). Offers medical, mental health, and social services by appointment and on a drop-in basis. Must be a patient of Tom Waddell to receive mental health treatment from an on-site psychiatrist. Includes a separate clinic for transgender people to receive primary care.

Tenderloin Outpatient Clinic (415) 673-5700

134 Golden Gate Avenue, San Francisco, CA 94102. www.hydestreetcs.org. Monday, Wednesday, Thursday, Friday: 9:00 a.m. to 5:00 p.m.; Tuesday: 9:00 a.m. to 2:00 p.m. Provides assessments, evaluation, psychotherapy, group therapy, and individual therapy on an appointment basis. Offers bilingual/bicultural services for the Arab/Muslim community.

Westside Crisis Clinic (415) 355-0311

245 11th Street, San Francisco, CA 94103. www.westside-health. org. Monday to Friday: 8:00 a.m.; Saturday: 9:00 a.m. A voluntary drop-in service open to any adult in need of emergency psychiatric care. Provides assessment, evaluation, crisis intervention, and stabilization services for people in a mental health crisis. Clients walk in, forming a line at 7:00 a.m. Hours extend until 6 p.m. or until appointments are finished.

EAST BAY

Asian Community Mental Health Services (510) 451-6729

310 8th Street, Suite 201, Oakland, CA 94607. www.achms.org. Provides assessment, evaluation, treatment, psycho-education, case management, substance use support, medication support, school-based programs, and youth programs.

Bay Area Children's Association (BACA) (510) 922-9757

111 Myrtle Street, Third Floor, Oakland, CA 94607. www.baca. org. An outpatient program for children and adolescents. Supports

---

Low, Medium, High Risk & Medical Emergency

Scales, measures, and methods vary in the conditions they define to represent low, medium, and high risk for suicide, while a medical emergency related to suicide risk is more consistent. Generally, suicide risk experts agree with the below classification.

• **Low risk**: Suicidal thoughts are present but the there is no preparation, plan, or intent.

• **Medium risk**: Suicidal thoughts are present with consideration of a plan. There is no concrete plan in place and no preparation or intent.

• **High risk**: A concrete plan has been developed with the intent to act in the near future.

• **Medical emergency**: An individual intends to attempt suicide immediately, within minutes or hours.

---

young people with acute risk of suicide. Offers patients ongoing dialogue around suicide and self-harm as well as weekly suicide risk assessments.

Crisis Support Services of Alameda County 1-800-309-2131

P.O. Box 3120, Oakland, CA 94609. www.crisissupport.org. Provides support groups and in-home counseling for elderly people in Alameda County with mental health challenges and risk of suicide. Also offers school-based counseling to youth in Alameda County struggling with the effects of trauma and violence in their communities.

La Cheim Behavioral Health Services (510) 596-8125

3031 Telegraph Avenue, Oakland, CA 94609. www.lacheim.org. A community alternative to hospitalization for people in need of intensive mental health support. Provides a comprehensive suicide intervention program. Capacity at La Cheim is limited and there is a waiting list for new clients.

Red Flags of High Risk

- Cogent plan
- Lethal means
- Near-term or imminent intent

La Clinica Casa del Sol (510) 535-6200

1501 Fruitvale Avenue, Oakland, CA 94601. www.laclinica.org. Monday to Thursday: 8:30 a.m. to 7:00 p.m. Friday: 8:30 a.m. to 6:00 p.m. Provides free, sliding-scale, and Covered California services to East Oakland residents in Spanish and English. Offers Wellness Recovery Action Planning (WRAP) groups, crisis intervention, and individual therapy.

The Hume Center (925) 825-1793

1333 Willow Pass Road, Suite 102, Concord, CA 94520. www.humecenter.org. An outpatient program for people at risk of hospitalization and for those who have recently been hospitalized. Provides support to people at moderate and low risk of suicide. Offers group therapy and individual therapy as well as medication support and education. Works to reduce the recidivism rate of people accessing inpatient hospitalization and to help create long-term care planning.

Native American Health Center (510) 535-4400

2950 International Boulevard, Oakland, CA 94601. beta.nativehealth.org. Monday to Friday: 9:00 a.m. to 5:00 p.m. A community clinic providing appointment-based assessment, evaluation, and crisis intervention services. Offers traditional healing, individual and group therapy, suicide prevention, and intervention support.

North County Crisis Clinic 1-800-491-9099

568 W. Grand Avenue, Oakland, CA 94621. Every day: 8:30 a.m. to 5 p.m. Works in collaboration with ACCESS to offer treatment to

mental health and substance abuse issues. Does not offer walk-ins, but appointments can be made by referral when calling ACCESS at (800) 491-9099 or Crisis Support Services of Alameda County at (800) 309-2131.

South County Crisis Response Program 1-800-491-9099

409 Jackson Street, Hayward, CA 94544. Monday to Friday: 8:30 a.m. to 5:00 p.m. A clinic and mobile response team that offers short-term outpatient services for 30 to 60 days. Appointments can be made by calling the ACCESS line: (800) 491-9099. Walk-ins are available.

Telecare's CHANGES (510) 553-8500

7200 Bancroft Avenue, Building B, Suite 133, Oakland, CA 94605. www.telecarecorp.com. A treatment center for adults ages 18 to 62 with a dual-diagnosis. Provides wraparound services as well as Level 2 intensive case management. Clients are referred to the program through ACCESS.

Telecare's Garfield Neurobehvioral Center (510) 261-9191

1451 28th Avenue, Oakland, CA 94601. www.telecarecorp.com. A treatment center for clients adults with primary neurobehavioral illnesses as well as mental health conditions. Services are geared toward building a client's personal sense of safety and wellness.

Telecare's STEPS (510) 238-5020

280 17th Street, Oakland, CA 94612. www.telecarecorp.com. A treatment center for adults with serious mental health conditions who are in need of short-term intensive case management. STEPS works closely with community partners to help reduce the recidivism of clients accessing intensive mental health services.

Telecare's STRIDES (510) 238-5020

280 17th Street, Oakland, CA 94612. www.telecarecorp.com. A treatment center for adults ages 18 to 62 with serious mental health conditions and risk of hospitalization. Works toward reducing this risk through psychotherapy, symptom management support, and care planning.

Diagnosis of Major Depression (DSM-5)

Five or more of the following symptoms present during the same 2-week period, representing a change from previous functioning. At least one symptom is either depressed mood or loss of interest or pleasure.

- Depressed mood as indicated by either subjective report or observation of others
- In children, irritability
- Markedly diminished interest or pleasure in activities
- Significant weight loss or significant change in appetite
- Insomnia or excess sleep
- Feelings of agitation or being slowed down observable by others
- Fatigue or loss of energy
- Feelings of worthlessness or excessive guilt
- Indecisiveness or diminished ability to think or concentrate
- Recurrent thoughts of death or suicidal ideation, a suicide attempt, or a specific plan for committing suicide

NORTH BAY

Children's Crisis Services (707) 253-4711

2344 Old Sonoma Road, Building D, Napa, CA 94559. www.countyofnapa.org. 24/7. Provides assessment, evaluation, intervention, and stabilization services to children and adolescents at risk of suicide.

Community Action Marin (415) 526-7500

3240 Kerner Boulevard, San Rafael, CA 94901. www.camarin.org A community organization providing peer support, crisis intervention, support for homeless populations, a crisis warm-line, and more. Offers WRAP groups. Community Action Marin's warm line can be accessed 24/7 at (415) 459-6330.

Mental Framework for Assessment & Management

When I first began to intensively study suicide risk assessment and management (A&M), I set out in pursuit of the holy grail. I was intent on finding a gold standard for A&M that would transform the complexity and messiness of suicide risk into a neat package I could tie up with a red bow. I've always been a good student. So I felt sure I could master suicide risk in the same way I mastered geometry and calculus.

Instead, the confusion deepened. I accumulated one book, scale, article, and academic protocol after another. In 2014 I traveled to the annual conference of the American Psychiatric Society at the Javits Center in New York City and, while there, attended 18 lectures and workshops on suicide risk. My stack of articles grew by four inches. My shelf of books expanded by three books. Still, the grail eluded me.

In the end, I concluded that suicide risk A&M has to be part of me. It's not something "out there" that does the work for me—a material thing I can lay my hands on physically. It's something in me—a "mental framework." Something in the consulting room triggers the framework, and then I gently and calmly take the patient into it. We *Talk About It*, calmly. I listen. I inquire. I assess. I manage as best I can. I listen more.

I often use paperwork as part of A&M, but the mental framework is the key thing. I encourage you to find your mental framework. Plunge into the articles and lectures, but don't seek out the holy grail. The grail is, in the end, your own confident framework and A&M style. The precise contours of that framework and style matter far less than simply having one.

Napa County Intensive Outpatient Program (707) 253-4063
2344 Old Sonoma Road, Building D, Napa, CA 94559. www.countyofnapa.org. An outpatient program providing crisis stabilization, 1-on-1 counseling, group counseling, and support around relapse and drug recovery. Services are available in both English and Spanish and are available in the morning and evening.

Sonoma County Indian Health Project (707) 521-4545

144 Stony Point Road, Santa Rosa, CA 95401. www.scihp.org. Monday to Friday: 8:00 a.m. to 5:00 p.m. Provides individual therapy, traditional healing, and crisis intervention. An on-call therapist is available for crisis intervention. Primarily for indigenous people, though open to all.

Telecare's Assertive
Community Treatment (ACT) (707) 568-2800

327 College Avenue, Santa Rosa, CA 95401. www.telecarecorp. com. A treatment center for people with serious mental health conditions in need of housing support, intensive case management, medication, and employment assistance. Referrals to this program are made through Sonoma County Mental Health.

PENINSULA

Adolescent Counseling Services (650) 424-0852

1717 Embarcadero Road, Suite 4000, Palo Alto, CA 94303. www. acs-teens.org. Offers on-site appointment-based services, including after-school counseling, adolescent substance use treatment, community education, and a queer youth group. Offers emergency intervention for clients at risk of suicide. Clients that cannot be seen immediately are referred to the PES at Mills Hospital.

Amen Clinic (650) 458-4615

1000 Marine Boulevard, Suite 100, Brisbane, CA 94005 www.amen-clinics.com. A treatment center for people with a variety of different mental health needs. Provides a multidisciplinary approach to healing through SPECT brain scans, personalized treatment plans, hormone replacement therapy, biomedical evaluations, and neurofeedback brain training.

Daly City Youth Center (650) 985-7000

2780 Junipero Serra Boulevard. Daly City, CA 94015. www.daly-cityyouth.org. Monday to Friday: 9:30 a.m. to 6:00 p.m. A youth

---

Elements of a Crisis Plan

- What will you *do* in a crisis (not *not do*)?
- Activities to diminish hopelessness, stress, agitation
- Relational safety net
- Access to clinician
- 911, emergency department

---

clinic that offers counseling services for coping with depression, bullying, anxiety, family problems, suicide ideation, and more. Offers same-day or next-day appointments.

Family and Children Services (650) 326-6576

375 Cambridge Avenue, Palo Alto, CA 94306. www.fcservices.org. A wraparound service provider for children, adolescents, and their families. Provides therapy, counseling, youth development services, queer youth services, substance use treatment, school based programing, and training. Family and Children Services does not offer walk-ins, but appointments can be made for the same or next week.

SOUTH BAY

Bay Area Children's Association (BACA)
San Jose (408) 996-7950

1175 Saratoga Avenue, Suite 14, San Jose, CA 95129. www.baca.org. An outpatient program supporting children and adolescents with low and moderate risk of suicide. Offers patients ongoing dialogue around suicide and self-harm as well as weekly suicide risk assessments.

Children's Shelter Mental Health Clinic (408) 558-5460

4525 Union Avenue, San Jose, CA 95124. www.php.com. An intensive outpatient clinic providing treatment services, crisis intervention, individual, group and family therapy, and psychotropic medication evaluation and treatment.

Community Solutions (408) 842-7138

9015 Murray Avenue, #100, Gilroy, CA 95020. www.communitysolutions.org. A wraparound service for youth and adults in Santa Clara County including therapy, crisis intervention, juvenile justice support, violence prevention programming, and re-entry programs.

East Valley Mental Health Center (408) 926-7950

1991 McKee Road, San Jose, CA 95116. Monday, Wednesday, Thursday, Friday: 8:00 a.m. to 5:00 p.m.; Tuesday: 8:00 a.m. to 8:00 p.m. Provides case management, crisis intervention, and medication consultations.

Las Plumas Mental Health Center (408) 272-6726

1650 Las Plumas Avenue, Suite K, San Jose, CA 95133. Monday to Thursday: 8:00 a.m. to 6:00 p.m.; Friday: 8:00 a.m. to 5:00 p.m. A community clinic that offers assessment, individual and family therapy, medication consultations, case management, and crisis intervention for adults ages 18 to 25. Services are accessed through the Santa Clara County Mental Health Call Center at 1-800-704-0900.

Momentum for Mental Health (408) 260-4040

438 North White Road, San Jose, CA 95127. www.momentumformentalhealth.org. A treatment center that offers intensive case management, crisis intervention, 1-on-1 therapy, and group therapy to people with serious mental health challenges.

Bay Area Suicide Statistics

- In the Bay Area region, there 7.51 to 10 suicides per 100,000 people.
- In San Francisco, there are 100 to 110 suicide deaths (45 to 48 homicides) in a population of 800,000.
- In 2013 the Golden Gate Bridge had the highest number of suicides on record with 46. There have been over 1,600 confirmed suicides on the Bridge since its construction.

CALMHSA and San Francisco Suicide Prevention, 2015

Stars Behavioral Health Group's
Starlight Community Services (408) 284-9000

1885 Lundy Avenue, Suite 223, San Jose, CA 95131. www.starsinc. com. A wraparound service for children and adolescents in San Jose providing therapy, psychotherapy, crisis intervention, juvenile justice support, and care planning.

10

Dialectical Behavioral Therapy

It is difficult to encapsulate the widespread wisdom of Dialectical Behavior Therapy (DBT) in the treatment of mental health disorders, including suicide risk, in a short space. Suffice it to say, DBT is one of the most powerful and enlightened psychotherapies to enter the field of behavioral health in the past half century. It is the only school of psychotherapy, at least as far as I am aware, specifically conceived and designed to treat acts of self-harm and suicidal behavior. For this reason, this chapter describes the core substance of DBT and provides more than two dozen referrals to DBT centers and DBT therapists in the Bay Area.

It is a common misconception that DBT is only instrumental in the treatment of self-cutting and other nonsuicidal self-harm behaviors. The old-fashion term for behaviors like these, whose intent may not be suicide at all, is "parasuicidal behaviors." Language changes frequently in the United States, and since the turn of the 21st century this terminology has fallen out of favor in preference to "nonsuicidal self-injurious behavior."

Nonsuicidal self-injurious behavior can be very complex. The best example is indeed self-cutting. One patient might self-cut as a distraction from emotional pain, displacing psychic pain to the physical body as a method of coping. Another patient may have a conception of self as "crazy" or "a freak," and somehow self-cutting symbolizes and reinforces this self-image. Another patient may be enacting self-hatred and a desire to self-punish in the behavior, and yet another may be enacting hatred and a desire to punish a parent, therapist, or other important figure in his or her life.

Self-cutting is very distressing to others. This may be another purpose of the act: to communicate distress and transfer it to another, perhaps with the hope that the other will provide solutions and relief. Nonsuicidal self-injurious behavior can also be a "cry for help," sometimes conscious, sometimes unconscious. Finally, self-cutting might be rooted in any of these underlying causes, *and* it might simultaneously reflect a desire to die or ambivalence about suicide and death.

What is certain is that a behavior like self-cutting is dangerous and concerning in 100% of cases. Even if the person cuts for motivations other than a desire to die, accidents happen, sudden impulses strike, and death may occur. Nonsuicidal self-injurious behavior should always be taken seriously and never dismissed as immature behavior or merely a "cry for help."

The structure of DBT is typically once or twice weekly individual psychotherapy supplemented by a weekly skills training group session, most commonly with another therapist. Whenever possible, family members are involved in the treatment. Additional support is provided, on a case-by-case basis.

DBT teaches patients four core sets of behavioral skills:

Distress Tolerance
How to tolerate pain in difficult situations, not change it

Mindfulness
The practice of being aware and present in the moment

Emotion Regulation
How to contain, soothe, and manage powerful emotions

Interpersonal Effectiveness
How to manage relationships, asking for what you want and saying no while maintaining self-respect

One overriding goal of DBT is impulse control. That is, the development of the capacity to observe powerful events happening inside the mind and body without relinquishing control to them. The impulse to self-cut is seen and appreciated but not followed. Likewise, a DBT patient comes to understand through mindfulness, distress tolerance, and emotional self-regulation that a suicidal death wish is an event occurring inside the mind as a function of an overwhelming mood state negatively coloring perceptions of the past, present, and future. These skills help a person restore a more accurate, broad, and integrated view of reality, disempowering the impulse from translating into self-destructive behaviors.

Most all DBT therapists treat nonsuicidal self-injurious behavior, and many treat active suicide risk as well, where there is clearly a fantasy or wish to die. It is okay to distinguish between nonsuicidal self-injurious behavior and "active suicidal ideation" or "active suicidal intent" when you call to make inquiries with DBT therapists. They know the difference—and comprehend the dangerous overlap between them—and will provide you with more information when you speak. If one DBT therapist's practice is not right for you, ask for referrals that better fit your needs.

SAN FRANCISCO

Center for Emotion Regulation Disorders (650) 539-8332
www.sfanxiety.com. Provides individual DBT for adults. Facilitated by Alexandria Murallo, Ph.D.

DBT at UCSF (415) 476-7227
401 Parnassus Avenue, San Francisco, CA 94143. www.psych.ucsf.edu. Provides group, individual, and family DBT. Specializes in DBT-A, adolescent issues, and depression.

Samantha Fordwood, Ph.D. (415) 963-3554
www.samanthafordwoodphd.com. Provides individual DBT for adolescents and adults as well as group DBT for adolescents.

Amanda Gale, Ph.D. (415) 295-1549
www.sfbaydbt.com. Provides individual DBT for adolescents and adults as well as group DBT for adolescents.

Anya Ho, Ph.D. (415) 505-3285
www.sfpsychology.com. Provides individual DBT for children, adolescents and adults.

Mindfulness Therapy Associates and Downtown DBT (415) 835-2164
870 Market Street, Suite 400, San Francisco, CA 94102. www.mindfulnesstherapy.org. Provides individual DBT for adolescents and adults as well as group DBT for adults. Specializes in eating disorders.

Shokooh Miry, Ph.D. (415) 298-0122
www.drmiry.com. Provides individual DBT for adolescents and adults as well as group DBT for eating disorders.

Jennifer Nam, Ph.D. (650) 323-5800 Ext. 2
www.drjennifernam.com. Provides individual DBT for adults.

Family & Friends
Talking About It Checklist

☐ Spent quiet time, with pen and paper, contemplating the loss of the person at risk of suicide.

☐ Asked a trusted friend, family member, or therapist for support and help in preparing.

☐ Prepared to directly ask if the person is having suicidal thoughts.

☐ Distilled your feelings into a loving message you wish to impart.

☐ Prepared to listen, empathize, and validate.

☐ Prepared referrals to professionals with same-day or next-day appointments.

☐ Prepared an emergency response plan.

See the "Family and Friends" section of the Introduction to this book and the spotlight titled, "Family and Friends: Preparing to Talk About It," for more in-depth and structured guidance on how to talk with someone who is at risk of suicide.

San Francisco DBT Center (415) 345-1396
1735-A Union Street, San Francisco, CA 94123. www.sfdbt.com. Provides individual DBT for adolescents and group DBT for adults. Offers meetings in Advanced Emotional Regularion and Skills-Based Therapy.

SF Bay DBT Collaborative (415) 779-6450
www.sfbaydbt.com. Provides group DBT for adults and sometimes for adolescents.

UCSF Young Adult and Family Center
DBT Program (415) 779-6450
www.psych.ucsf.edu. Provides individual and group DBT for adolescents and adults. Offers groups for families and graduates.

Ongoing Assessment

Continue to monitor suicidal ideation at every session, no matter how well the therapy appears to be progressing, until it is clear that the patient is no longer having any suicidal ideation.

Shea, The Practical Art of Suicide Assessment, 2011

EAST BAY

Clearwater Counseling
and Assessment Services (510) 596-8137

345 38th Street, Oakland, CA 94609. www.clearwaterclinic.com. Provides individual and goup DBT for children, adolescents, adults, and families. Specializes in eating disorders and substance use disorders.

East Bay Behavior Therapy Center (925) 956-4636

Walnut Creek, CA. www.eastbaybehaviortherapycenter.com. Provides individual and group DBT for adolescents and adults. Offers group DBT for families.

Amanda Gale, Ph.D. (415) 295-1549

Orinda, CA. www.sfbaydbt.com. Provides individual DBT for adolescents and adults as well as group DBT for adults.

Mt. Diablo Psychological Services (925) 699-3476

91 Gregory Lane, Suite 19, Pleasant Hill, CA 94523. www.mtdiablopsychologicalservices.com. Provides individual and group DBT for adolescents, adults, and families.

Oakland DBT and Mindfulness Center (510) 239-5698

5767 Broadway, Suite 101, Oakland, CA 94618. www.oaklanddbtcenter.com. Provides individual and group DBT for adolescents, adults, and couples. Offers group DBT for families.

Questions to Probe for Preparation for Suicide

- If you were to commit suicide, what steps would you take in advance of the actual act of ending your life?
- Have you taken any steps (online research, obtaining means, drafting a will, saying goodbye, writing a suicide note)?
- Have you ever written a suicide note? Thought about writing a suicide note? What would you say in the note?

Katherine Schultz LCSW (925) 465-7474

Orinda, CA 94618. www.katherineschulz.com. Provides individual and group meetings for adults.

NORTH BAY

Center for Innovative DBT (415) 339-8001 Ext. 1

45 San Clemente Drive, C 200, Corte Madera, CA 94925. www. InnovativeDBT.com. Provides individual and group DBT for adolescents and families. Offers group DBT for friends.

DBT Center of Marin (415) 459-5206

895 Sir Francis Drake Boulevard, San Anselmo, CA 94960. www. dbtmarin.com. Provides individual and group DBT for adolescents and adults. Offers group DBT for parents, families, and friends.

Family Service Agency of Marin (415) 491-5728

San Rafael and Sausalito, CA. www.fsamarin.org. Provides individual DBT for adolescents and adults as well as group DBT for adults.

Annette Holloway, Psy.D. (415) 843-1453

San Anselmo, CA. www.familytherapysf.com. Provides individual DBT for adults.

PENINSULA

Sarah Adler, Psy.D. (650) 468-0771
Palo Alto, CA. www.paloaltopsychologygroup.com. Provides individual DBT for adults.

Jason Angel, Ph.D. (650) 323-5800
Palo Alto, CA. www.paloaltopsychologygroup.com. Provides individual DBT for adolescents and adults.

California DBT Peninsula Associates (650) 917-9100
329 S. San Antonio Road, Suite 3, Los Altos, CA 94022. www.californiadbt.com. Provides individual and group DBT for adolescents and adults. Has locations in Belmont, Los Altos, and Redwood City.

Sara Landes, Ph.D. (650) 323-5800 Ext. 2
Menlo Park, CA. Sara.landes@va.gov. Provides individual DBT for female vetrans.

Marilyn Foley, Ph.D. (650) 634-9896
Redwood City, CA. Mjfoley9@gmail.com. Provides individual and group DBT for adolescents and adults as well as group DBT for family and friends.

Mid Peninsula DBT/ Mary F. Reed, M.F.T. (650) 996–4618
617 Veterans Boulevard, Suite 212, Redwood City, CA 94063. Provides group, individual and phone DBT for adolescents, adults, couples, and families.

Mid Peninsula DBT/ Tami Schmalz, M.F.T. (650) 996–4618
617 Veterans Boulevard, Suite 212, Redwood City, CA 94063. Provides group, individual, and phone DBT for adolescents and families.

Mid Peninsula DBT/ Helen Selenati, M.F.T. (650) 596-0807
617 Veterans Boulevard, Suite 212, Redwood City, CA 94063. www.midpeninsuladbt.com. Provides group, individual, and phone DBT for adolescents and adults.

The Role of Suffering in "Suicidal Gestures"

So often I am asked by clinicians and family members about the challenge of two distinct types of suicide risk: "real" suicide risk vs. "cries for help," "manipulation," or "acting out" in which there may be suicidal statements and behaviors but no apparent true suicidal intent. The former often elicits sympathy and concern in others, while the latter may engender these same feelings in combination with perplexity, frustration, and anger.

The often impulsive behaviors characterized as "cries for help" have been described for decades in the psychiatric literature as "suicidal gestures," as distinguished from suicide attempts in which there is, to some degree, a wish to die. An essential concept to understand in all human psychology and some suicidal behaviors is that of "secondary gain." When behaviors are motivated in part by secondary gain it means that interpersonal or social advantages attend to the behavior, such as an increase in attention or sympathy from others or the forestalling of a breakup or other loss. This motivation, it is important to recognize, may be conscious or entirely unconscious.

Be assured that suicidal behavior is complex. It can be extremely confusing to health professionals, family members, and friends. What unites the entire spectrum of suicidal thoughts, feelings, and behaviors, however, is the internal experience of suffering.

When you *Talk About It*, do not rush to identify or uncover motivations like secondary gain. Do not rush to label a behavior as a "suicidal gesture." Rather, leave these interpretations aside and appreciate the depth of suffering. Empathize with the suffering. Seek to understand the suffering. Stay with care and concern for the suffering. Seek help to attend to the suffering.

Jennifer Nam, Ph.D. (650) 323-5800 Ext. 2

Palo Alto, CA. www.drjennifernam.com. Provides individual DBT for adults.

Silicon Valley DBT (408) 345-5070

Los Altos, CA. www.siliconvalleydbt.com. Provides individual and group DBT for adolescents, adults, and couples. Offers group DBT for families and friends.

Stanford University DBT Program (650) 498-9111

Palo Alto, CA. Provides individual and group DBT for adolescents and adults. Offers group DBT for families and those with bipolar disorder, conversion disorder, and eating disorder. The above number is for Adult Intake. For Adolescent Intake, call (650) 723-5511.

Christy Telch, Ph.D. (650) 323-1637

Palo Alto, CA. Provides individual DBT for adults with eating disorders.

SOUTH BAY

Melinda Carlisle Brackett, L.M.F.T. (408) 893-4032

San Jose, CA. www.southbaydbt.com. Provides individual DBT for adults and group DBT for adults and couples.

California Bay Area DBT
San Jose and Silicon Valley (408) 893-4032

991 West Heading Street, Suite #106, San Jose, CA 95126. www.southbaydbt.com. Provides group DBT for adults ages 19 and up. Specializes in eating disorders and substance use disorders.

Crestwood Center San Jose (408) 275-1010

1425 Fruitdale Avenue, San Jose, CA 95128. www.crestwoodbehavioralhealth.com. Provides inpatient and residential DBT for adolescents, adults, and families. Locations in Angwin, Vallejo, Sunnyvale, and Stockton.

Suggestions on How to Improve This Book?

Please contact me and share your thoughts. Email info@merritt-mentalhealth.com or call 415-285-3774.

Caroline C. Fleck, Ph.D. (425) 200-5425
San Jose, CA. www.drcarolinefleck.com. Provides individual DBT for adolescents and adults.

Hooria Jazaieri, M.F.T. (408) 462-1447
San Jose, CA. www.outlookCBT.com. Provides individual DBT for adolescents and adults.

Sanguine Counseling
and In-the-Moment DBT Program (408) 676-7081
1769 Park Ave, Suite 210, San Jose, CA, 95126. www.sanguinecounseling.com. Provides individual and group DBT for adolescents and adults.

Silicon Valley DBT (408) 345-5070
San Jose, CA. www.siliconvalleydbt.com. Provides individual and group DBT for adolescents, adults, and couples. Offers group DBT for families and friends.

11

Adolescent & Youth Services

Nothing motivates me more in all aspects of my clinical and consulting work than the health and well-being of children and adolescents. Nothing motivates me more in my suicide prevention work than keeping children and adolescents alive.

This principle of "safety first" is one reason clinicians must be solid at suicide risk assessment and management. If there is a whiff of risk, the clinician must hold on and go deeper. The clinician must *Talk About It*, calmly and persistently, until relative safety has been established. The clinician must understand what a Safety Plan, or Crisis Response Plan, is and know how to implement one collaboratively with every patient at risk .

Suicide risk is like angina—classic condition of heart pain due to blockage of coronary arteries. No matter what it takes, the clinician assessing a cardiac patient must determine whether the blockage is "stable" or "unstable"—with a "low risk" of imminent heart attack or a "high risk." Until this is known, there's really little else of importance to talk about in the clinical encounter. Unstable angina is life-threatening.

My goal is to aid every patient and family to achieve "low risk" for suicide in the same way cardiologists examine patients, perform procedures, and prescribe dietary changes, exercise, and medications until they feel convinced that there is low risk of heart attack.

I recommend this high standard to colleagues, and the best way to achieve it is continuous lifelong education in suicide risk assessment and management. As I have said elsewhere in these pages, the first ten to fifteen hours of learning is the hardest. Then there is joy in the learning and great satisfaction in the work. Your anxiety diminishes. You feel more confident and competent. You know how to listen, what to say, what to assess, what to do, where to turn, where to go. Families benefit. Patients benefit. Possibly, you save lives.

To me, there is something unique about the life of a child, adolescent, or young adult. The reason is that the fifteen year old, the eighteen year old, and the twenty-two year old have not yet had the chance to live. In the context of a psychiatric or addictive illness, something goes wrong in the life of a young person—in society, school, family, friendships, or romantic relationships—and, following this, a distorted, impulsive suicidal state of mind sets in. Then, in some cases, death occurs.

More than once, I have been a participant in conversations about rational suicide. I can't say that I am a fan or advocate of rational suicide in any age group—suicide due to intractable pain, physical disability, mental disability, or lack of quality of life—but it's fair to say that, philosophically and ethically, there are complex arguments worth voicing in the case of some adults with unrelenting, long-term suffering and pain with little time left and little chance of restoration of quality of life.

The same simply cannot be said about the life of a young person. Youth suicide is tragic—always tragic, with no room for debate about existential philosophy, the relief of suffering, or poor quality of life. For this reason, my greatest passion of all in suicide prevention is youth. I believe that all young people, without exception, have the capacity to heal emotionally and to develop meaningful, relationship-rich lives. First, they have to stay alive.

Only then can they and their families get into the right treatment and benefit from it.

The resources in this chapter are diverse. They range from Crisis Stabilization Units to Clinics to Residential Programs. They are resources you can access at various hours, day and night. There are people on the other side of the telephone line who will answer your questions, help you strategize, and teach you how to approach an adolescent or youth you are concerned about. Pick up the phone. Get started now. Take out time to get empowered to *Talk About It* with a young person who is in crisis and possibly at risk of suicide.

SAN FRANCISCO

Comprehensive Child Crisis Service (415) 970-3800
3801 3rd Street, Stuite 400, San Francisco, CA 94124. www.sfdph. org. A crisis intervention service for children and adolescents in San Francisco. Provides 30 days of ongoing stabilization and crisis management for approved clients.

Edgewood Center for Children and Families (415) 969-4135
1801 Vicente Street, San Francisco, CA 94116. www.edgewood.org. An organization providing crisis stabilization services, hospital diversion services, intensive mental health support in the IOP and PHP levels, and school-based programming.

Huckleberry Youth Services (415) 668-2622
3310 Geary Boulevard, San Francisco, CA 94118. www.huckle-berryyouth.org. Monday, Tuesday, Wednesday, Friday: 9:00 a.m. to 5:00 p.m.; Thursday: 2:00 p.m. to 6:00 p.m. A clinic providing assessment on appointment and drop-in basis as well as evaluation and crisis intervention. Serves adolescents and adults ages 11 to 24 living in San Francisco.

Larkin Street Youth Services (415) 673-0911
134 Golden Gate Avenue, San Francisco, CA 94102. www.larkin-streetyouth.org. Monday, Wednesday, Thursday, Friday: 9:00 a.m. to 5:00 p.m.; Tuesday: 11:00 a.m. to 5:00 p.m. A clinic providing assessment, evaluation, and crisis intervention to homeless youth and adults ages 11 to 24 living in San Francisco.

San Francisco Suicide Prevention (415) 984-1900
P.O. Box 191350, San Francisco, CA 94119. www.sfsuicide.org. The nation's oldest suicide hotline and a leader in suicide prevention services and strategies. Provides crisis support hotline, texting, and chat. Offers education in workplaces, churches, organizations, and small groups. Support groups are available for people who have survived a suicide attempt. Risk reduction programs are available for youth. More information in the Broad-Based Suicide Prevention, Hotlines, Advocacy, and Education & Trainings chapters.

Family and Friends
Advice to Parents from Adam Strassberg, M.D.

In March of 2015 Silicon Valley psychiatrist Dr. Adam Strassberg responded to a teen suicide occurring one week earlier in Palo Alto by publishing an online article in *The Palo Alto Weekly*. The death of a 15-year-old high school student was part of a cluster of youth suicides on nearby Caltrain tracks. The piece, entitled "Keep Calm and Parent On: What Can Parents Do Right Now to Decrease the Risk of Suicide in their Children?" went viral.

Within weeks the insightful article received more than 150,000 hits and soon became a catalyst for national dialogue on adolescent suicide and American culture, most notably the high-pressure culture of Silicon Valley. Dr. Strassberg provides valuable counsel to parents worried about suicide risk in high school aged youth. For this reason I am sharing his short list of seven suggestions to help parents "Keep Calm and Parent On":

1. Make your teen sleep
2. Talk with your teen
3. Model mental health treatment for your teen
4. Want the best for your child, not for your child to be the best
5. It's you and the teachers versus your teen, not you and your teen versus the teachers
6. Get a pet
7. Keep calm

In his own words Dr. Strassberg underscores the main theme of this book—*Talk About It*. In his section "Talk with your teen," he reminds us that asking about suicide does not increase the risk of suicide. That is mythology. Asking does not plant ideas in a person's mind. On the contrary, it decreases the risk by opening dialogue. "So please," Strassberg says, "do ask your teen directly about suicide."

Other crucial take-home messages from the article are the importance of modeling emotional expression and seeking professional help in the family and, vitally, loving kids for who they are, not what you hope they will become.

Continued

On modeling, he urges parents not to hide their true selves from their children. Instead, discuss your feelings and share your vulnerabilities openly: "If you are sad, if you are unhappy, talk with your spouse, friends, and family about your feelings. Let your children see you cry, let them see you laugh, let them see you touch, hold, and comfort one another. Most of all, if you are suffering from depression or any other psychological difficulties, let them see you seek appropriate professional treatment. If you and your spouse are having marital difficulties, let them see you both enter couples counseling."

Regarding love over achievement, Strassberg concludes with a memorable metaphor. "The 'Koala Dad' is the far better parent than the 'Tiger Mom.'" His advice is "more sleep, more free unscheduled time to play and to grow, less homework, more balance, and better stress tolerance."

If you are concerned about a teen, reach out and ask for help. *Talk About It* with trusted others and with your teen. You can read more of Dr. Strassberg's advice and over 100 posts by parents on *The Palo Alto Weekly* website.

EAST BAY

Bay Area Children's Association (BACA) (510) 922-9757

111 Myrtle Street, Third Floor, Oakland, CA 94607. www.baca.org. An outpatient program for children and adolescents. Supports young people with acute risk of suicide. Offers patients ongoing dialogue around suicide and self-harm as well as weekly suicide risk assessments.

Crisis Support Services of Alameda County 1-800-260-0094

P.O. Box 3120, Oakland, CA 94609. A county service providing a comprehensive youth suicide prevention program called Teens 4 Life, which is a suicide prevention program that educates students, teachers, and school mental health professionals about suicide and suicide risk.

East Bay Agency for Children PALS Program (510) 531-7551
303 Van Buren Avenue, Oakland, CA 94610. www.ebac.org. An in-school counseling program offered to low-income students. Provides 1-on-1 counseling, suicide assessments, and interventions when necessary.

Familiy, Youth and Children's Services
of Berkeley and Albany (510) 981-5280
3282 Adeline Street, Berkeley, CA 94704. www.ci.berkeley.ca.us. An organization providing intensive crisis stabilization and mental health support services including outpatient counseling to youth and adolescents.

La Clinica Casa del Sol (510) 535-6200
1501 Fruitvale Avenue, Oakland, CA 94601. www.laclinica.org. A clinic providing free, sliding-scale, and Covered California services to East Oakland residents in Spanish and English. Offers Wellness Recovery Action Planning (WRAP) groups, crisis intervention, and individual therapy.

Telecare's Willow Rock Center (510) 895-5502
2050 Fairmont Drive, San Leandro, CA. 94578 www.telecarecorp.com. A walk-in crisis stabilization unit and an inpatient psychiatric facility for children and adolescents. Clients are referred to Willow

---

Hotlines for Youth

California

California Youth Crisis Line 1-800-843-5200

Teen Crisis Text Line Text "START" to 741741

The Trevor Project Lifeline 1-866-488-7386

Bay Area

Huckleberry Youth House Crisis 24-Hour Hotline (415) 621-2929

Child & Adolescent Hotline and Prevention Program (650) 567-5437

Rock either by the police, an emergency department, an outpatient program, or on a self-referral basis. Willow Rock Center offers suicide assessments for all clients as well as detailed care planning for people who do not need inpatient hospitalization. Outpatient services are available at Willow Rock until a more appropriate longer-term facility is located. **Note:** East Bay youth at risk of suicide are most likely to be transferred to Willow Rock from an emergency department. Youth in need of hospitalization should go here first.

NORTH BAY

Children's Crisis Services (707) 253-4711
2344 Old Sonoma Road, Building D, Napa, CA 94559. www.countyofnapa.org. A mental health program providing crisis services to children and adolescents. Offers assessment, intervention, and stabilization services to children at suicide risk or serious mental distress.

Huckleberry Youth Programs (415) 258-4944
361 Third Street, Suite G, San Rafael, CA 94901. www.huckleberryyouth.org. A clinic providing assessment on appointment and drop-in basis as well as evaluation and crisis intervention. Serves adolescents and adults.

Muir Woods Adolescent and Family Services (415) 299-6268
1733 Skillman Lane, Petaluma, CA 94952. www.muirwoodteen.com. A boys residential treatment center in Sonoma County and coed outpatient treatment center in Marin County.

Youth Suicide 2015 CDC Report

Youth suicide is a growing national concern. As documented in the following 2015 report of the Centers of Disease Control (CDC), approximately 157,000 youth receive medical care in Emergency Departments in the United States for self-inflicted injuries each year, and some 4,600 young people die of suicide annually.

From the report:

Suicide is a serious public health problem that affects even young people. For youth between the ages of 10 and 24, suicide is the third leading cause of death. It results in approximately 4600 lives lost each year. The top three methods used in suicides of young people include firearm (45%), suffocation (40%), and poisoning (8%).

Deaths from youth suicide are only part of the problem. More young people survive suicide attempts than actually die. A nationwide survey of youth in grades 9–12 in public and private schools in the United States (U.S.) found that 16% of students reported seriously considering suicide, 13% reported creating a plan, and 8% reporting trying to take their own life in the 12 months preceding the survey. Each year, approximately 157,000 youth between the ages of 10 and 24 receive medical care for self-inflicted injuries at Emergency Departments across the U.S.

Suicide affects all youth, but some groups are at higher risk than others. Boys are more likely than girls to die from suicide. Of the reported suicides in the 10 to 24 age group, 81% of the deaths were males and 19% were females. Girls, however, are more likely to report attempting suicide than boys. Cultural variations in suicide rates also exist, with Native American/Alaskan Native youth having the highest rates of suicide-related fatalities. A nationwide survey of youth in grades 9–12 in public and private schools in the U.S. found Hispanic youth were more likely to report attempting suicide than their black and white, non-Hispanic peers.

CDC, 2015

Advice to Health Professionals

The importance of clinical consultation cannot be overstated.

Jobes, 2006

PENINSULA

Adolescent Counseling Services (650) 424-0852

1717 Embarcadero Road Suite 4000, Palo Alto, CA 94303. www. acs-teens.org. A clinic offering on-site appointment-based services, including after-school counseling, adolescent substance use treatment, community education, and a queer youth group. Offers emergency intervention for clients at risk of suicide. Clients that cannot be seen immediately are referred to the PES at Mills Hospital.

Daly City Youth Center (650) 985-7000

2780 Junipero Serra Boulevard, Daly City, CA 94015. www.dalycityyouth.org. A youth clinic that offers counseling services for coping with depression, bullying, anxiety, family problems, suicidal ideation, and more. Offers same-day or next-day appointments.

Edgewood Center for
Children and Families IOP (415) 969-4135

957 Industrial Road, Suite B, San Carlos, CA 94070. www.edgewood.org. A treatment center for children and adolescents ages 6 to 14. Provides crisis stabilization and long-term planning to reduce high-risk behaviors.

Family and Children Services (650) 326-6576

375 Cambridge Avenue, Palo Alto, CA 94306. www.fcservices.org. A wraparound service provider for children, adolescents, and their families. Provides therapy, counseling, youth development services, queer youth services, substance use treatment, school based programing, and training. Family and Children Services does not offer walk-ins, but appointments can be made for the same or next week.

SOUTH BAY

Bay Area Children's Association (BACA)
San Jose (408) 996-7950
1175 Saratoga Avenue, Suite 14, San Jose, CA 95129. www.baca.org. An outpatient program supporting children and adolescents with low and moderate risk of suicide. Offers patients ongoing dialogue around suicide and self-harm as well as weekly suicide risk assessments.

Community Solutions (408) 842-7138
9015 Murray Avenue, #100, Gilroy, CA 95020. www.communitysolutions.org. A wraparound service for youth and adults in Santa Clara County including therapy, crisis intervention, juvenile justice support, violence prevention programming, and re-entry programs.

EMQ Families First Crisis Stabilization Unit (408) 364-4083
251 Llewellyn Avenue, Campbell, CA 95008. WWW.emqff.org. A 24/7 crisis intervention service for children and adolescents in Santa Clara County.

Project Cornerstone (408) 351-6482
80 Saratoga Avenue, Santa Clara, CA 95051. www.projectcornerstone.org. An organization providing youth-focused trainings to organizations, schools, youth, and the community. Trainings include bully prevention programs.

Youth Suicide Risk Research Project

Merritt Mental Health is launching an initiative called the "Youth Suicide Risk Research Project." The purpose of this initiative is to investigate and document evidence-based strategies for identifying and treating youth suicide risk.

Sign up for news on the Merritt Mental Health website under "Mental Health Compass." To share ideas or collaborate, please email info@merrittmentalhealth.com.

NATIONAL

Crisis Text Line Text "START" to 741741
A hotline providing text message crisis support.

Half of Us www.halfofus.org
An online project of the Jed Foundation providing mental health and suicide risk information and resources for college students. Provides information to those in need as well as friends of those in need regarding how to tell signs of suicide risk and where to get help.

The Jed Foundation (212) 647-7544
6 East 39th Street, Suite 1204, New York, NY 10016. www.jedfoundation.org. A national organization dedicated to promoting emotional health and preventing suicide among college and university students. Collaborates with mtvU on halfofus.com, which uses stories of students and high-profile artists to increase awareness about mental health problems and the importance of getting help. Runs the ULifeline.org online mental health support network.

Lifeline Crisis Chat www.suicidepreventionlifeline.org
A hotline providing live Internet chat to help reduce stress and increase feelings of empowerment.

The Trevor Project Lifeline 1-866-488-7386
A hotline providing support for LGBTQ youth, ages 13-24. Calls go to LA or NYC.

ULifeline www.ulifeline.org
An online project of the Jed Foundation providing mental health and suicide risk information and resources for college students. Provides resources to those in need as well as their friends. Offers an online suicide risk self-evaluation.

12

Education & Training

Nothing matters more in suicide prevention than basic education for health professionals, educators, civil servants, family members, and friends. The first skill to be learned is sensitive compassionate listening. The second is gentle probing to understand if there are suicidal thoughts and, if so, the nature of them. One way to order a screening or brief assessment is a stepwise exploration of 1) ideation 2) methods 3) plan 4) intent and 5) imminence. Are there suicidal thoughts? Are the thoughts passive wishes to die or active wishes to take one's own life? How would others feel and react to the suicide? Is there a plan, intent, and, if so, a timeline? What are the risk factors and protective factors?

A third vital component of suicide prevention is preparedness. Having this book on hand is one form of preparedness. It is tangible. It reminds you of methods and procedures and provides immediate resources that enable you to reach out to others for advice and help in a matter of seconds. Remember to *Talk About It*. Make a phone call. Too often family members and professionals allow fears and uncertainties to grip and paralyze them, when assistance and guidance are only a phone call away.

You can always read online. There are a dozen excellent websites offering instruction and assessment tools. Peruse them. Take notes. However, there is no replacement for human contact when we are suffering anxiety and fear. Do not stop at online research or reading this book. Call and speak to others and keep speaking to them until you have a plan in place that gives you a feeling of security and safety.

One part of preparedness is knowing your next step if brief assessment reveals suicide risk. If there is no risk—no suicidal ideation past or present, minimal risk factors, and numerous protective factors—no further steps are necessary. If there is low risk, what is your plan? Moderate risk? High or imminent risk?

No family member is an island. No doctor, therapist, or teacher is an island. We all need help from others. In each of these risk categories, what will you do and to whom will you turn for help? What will you recommend to your loved one, patient, or student? Do you have an emergency plan ready? Mobile crisis number handy? Have you identified an emergency department near you? How will you get there? If you are a family member or friend who has decided to *Talk About It* with someone you are concerned about, have you found a qualified doctor or therapist in advance and confirmed availability for an appointment?

These seem to be many challenging questions—made all the more daunting by our fragmented, labyrinthine mental health system—but answering them and becoming prepared, in fact, is only a matter of investing time and energy into the project. There are three chief steps to take: 1) understand the basics of suicide risk assessment and management 2) know your local resources and 3) link them together into systematic action plans based on risk stratification.

This book helps with all three of these steps, but clinicians have to do more legwork. First, figure our your own method of assessment and management. There are many to choose from. Personalize your method. It has to feel right and come natural to you. Second, locate yourself on the map and think through specific scenarios based on local hotlines, mobile crisis units, emergency departments, hospitals, clinics, colleagues, and programs. Create a file with your plans, or outline your plans on the blank pages at the end of this book.

Finally, there is no better way to prepare and learn skills than by participating in a workshop or training. It's a great way to spend a half-day or day. In a workshop you can *Talk About It* with the laser-sharp aim of developing or improving your system for assessment and management. This chapter contains the names and contact information of more than a dozen Bay Area organizations offering trainings. Call each individually to learn more. Sign up and attend the one you feel best fits your particular circumstances and needs.

SAN FRANCSICO

Mental Health Association of San Francisco (415) 421-2926
Flood Building, 870 Market St #928, San Francisco, CA 94102. www.mentalhealthsf.org. Offers WRAP training as well as other trainings throughout the year.

Merritt Mental Health (415) 285-3774
3786 20th Street, San Francisco, CA 94110. www.merrittmental-health.com. Merritt Mental Health plans to launch workshops and trainings. Check the website for more information or call the office number above.

San Francisco State University
1600 Holloway Avenue, San Francisco, CA 94132 . www.sfsu.edu. Offers ASIST trainings. Contact Susan Chen at susachen@sfsu.edu.

San Francisco Suicide Prevention (415) 984-1900
P.O. Box 191350, San Francisco, CA 94119. www.sfsuicide.org. Offers school-based crisis intervention trainings as well as suicide prevention education in workplaces, churches, organizations, and small groups.

EAST BAY

Contra Costa Crisis Center (925) 939-1916
307 Lennon Lane, Walnut Creek, CA 94598. www.crisis-center.org. Offers ASIST trainings.

Crisis Support Services of Alameda County (510) 420-2460
P.O. Box 3120, Oakland, CA 94609. www.crisissupport.org. Offers suicide assessment and intervention trainings for gatekeepers as well as mental health consultation trainings, mental health first aid, and a comprehensive youth suicide prevention program called Teens 4 Life, which is a suicide prevention program that educates students, teachers, and school mental health professionals about suicide and suicide risk. Trains mental health interns to do counseling in Alameda County schools.

The Hume Center (925) 825-1793

1333 Willow Pass Road, Suite 102, Concord, CA 94520. www. humecenter.org. Offers training program for practicum students, pre-doctoral interns, post-doctoral fellows, and other behavioral health care professionals, with some trainings involving suicide prevention.

Crucial Link
Suicide Risk and Substance Use Disorders

There are numerous risk factors for suicide, including previous suicide attempt, a family history of suicide, depression, bipolar disorder, recent loss, and hopelessness, among others.

However, no risk factor is so underrecognized and underappreciated worldwide as alcohol and drug abuse and intoxication. On the one hand, substances are widely deployed to stanch the discomfort and pain of grief, depression, anxiety, and other mental conditions. While they do achieve transient anesthetic and anxiolytic effects in this regard, they do vastly more than this to the sensitive brain. Substances, ingested heavily or routinely as a primary means of coping with life's interpersonal and social challenges, staunch human development.

The result is that a 30, 40, or 50 year-old who began abusing substances in this way at age 15, persisting in the abuse over the years, becomes trapped at the developmental age of 15. When he or she is "failing" in adult life, the person is often fiercely self-critical and self-blaming. Not infrequently, these intense feelings of being stuck and failing spur hopelessness and explorations of suicide as a solution. In fact, though, what is truly to blame for the deflation and paralysis? The substances.

The substances put a halt to the emotional growth of the addicted person. Of course he or she cannot cope with adult life or adult life crisis. That's a very tough thing to do at a persisting developmental age of 15 guided by a brain still seeped in substances.

The way out is not suicide. The way out is to stop the substances, rekindling human emotional development and maturation with

Continued

all its ups and downs, joys, griefs, and inevitable growing pains.

Thus one way substances contribute to suicide risk is through this mechanism of arrested development, triggering grief, depression, paralysis, and self-blame. Another is emotional and behavioral disinhibition due to acute intoxication. Many people attempt or commit suicide while drunk or high.

Substances make us lose our senses while, paradoxically, boosting our confidence and convictions. The result of this depressed, overdetermined state of mind can be suicide. Research bears out this tight association between substance use disorders and suicide risk. More than 50% of individuals have used alcohol or other drug just before a suicide attempt (American Psychiatric Association, Practice Guideline for the Assessment and Treatment of Patients with Suicidal Behaviors, 2003).

In the 2013 National Survey on Drug Use and Health, investigators found that substance use disorders were consistently linked with far higher rates of suicidal ideation, planning, and attempts than those without substance disorders. In this survey, individuals aged 18 or older with a past year substance use disorder were almost four times as likely to have had serious thoughts of suicide in the past year (11.4 vs. 3.2 percent). They also made suicide plans more than four times as often (4.2 vs.0.9 percent) and were almost six times as likely to have attempted suicide (2.3 vs. 0.4 percent) (2013 National Survey on Drug Use and Health, U.S Department of Health and Human Services).

Further, abuse of substances, including alcohol, is the second most frequently found risk factor for suicide, after mood disorder. And substance use disorders are particularly common in adolescents and young adults who die by suicide (APA, Practice Guideline, 2003). None of these studies take in consideration fatal drug overdose, which in many cases may be unreported suicides and run at approximately 43,000 per year (2002-2013 National Survey on Drug Use and Health, CDC 2015).

Never underestimate the impact of substance abuse and dependence as a risk factor for suicide. Talk about suicide risk *and* talk about substance abuse and intoxication. Too often, substances and mood disorders make for a lethal combination.

NORTH BAY

The Crisis, Assessment, Prevention, and Education (CAPE) Team (707) 565-3542

Santa Rosa, CA. www.sonoma-county.org. Offers Know the Signs trainings for peers and parents.

Marin Teen Mental Health Board (415) 272-5123

317 Scenic Road, Fairfax, CA 94930. john@iheartcasey.com. Offers education and training about suicide and depression for Marin county high school students and their parents.

North Bay Suicide Prevention Project (415) 499-1193 Ext. 3004

San Rafael, CA. www.fsamarin.org. Offers ASIST, QPR, safeTALK, and AMSR trainings.

PENINSULA

Adolescent Counseling Services (650) 424-0852

1717 Embarcadero Road, Suite 4000, Palo Alto, CA 94303. www.acs-teens.org. Offers community education events. A "99 Tips for Talking with Your Teenager" brochure is available on their website in both English and Spanish.

Kara (650) 321-5272

457 Kingsley Avenue, Palo Alto, CA 94301. www.kara-grief.org. Offers training for professional caregivers and first responders as well as workshops to community organizations like faith groups, senior groups, schools, and the general public.

Palo Alto Therapy (650) 461-9026

407 Sherman Avenue, Palo Alto, CA 94306. www.paloaltotherapy.com. A group practice that offers QPR trainings.

Protective Factors

- Strong connections to family, friends, or community
- Hope for the future
- Effective mental health care
- Strong therapeutic relationship with a mental health professional
- Strong help-seeking skills
- Self-efficacy in problem solving
- Cultural or religious beliefs that discourage or prohibit suicide
- Attachment to life
- Responsibility to family members, friends, pets, or life mission
- Perception of negative impact of suicide on loved ones
- Willingness to follow a Crisis Plan

Project Safety Net (650) 463-4928

4000 Middlefield Road, Palo Alto, CA 94306. www.psnpaloalto. com. Organizes education opportunities in the community. Maintains a list of local suicide prevention education and training opportunities on their Events page: www.psnpaloalto.com/events

San Mateo County's Behavioral Health and Recovery Services Department (650) 573-2541

225 West 37th Avenue, San Mateo, CA 94403. www.smhealth.org/ BHRS. Offers ASIST trainings, Crisis Intervention Training (CIT), SMART, and Mental Health First Aid. Mental Health First Aid is geared toward adults and youth and includes sections that focus on suicide prevention.

Star Vista (650) 591-9623

610 Elm Street, Suite 212, San Carlos, CA 94070. www.star-vista. org. Offers trainings for hotline and crisis counselors as well as suicide prevention presentations for the local community.

SOUTH BAY

Living Hope (408) 398-7071
San Jose, CA. www.livinghopesps.com. Offers ASIST, safeTALK, and suicideTALK trainings. Online registration available.

Project Cornerstone (408) 351-6482
Santa Clara, CA. www.projectcornerstone.org. Offers youth-focused trainings to organizations, schools, youth, and the community. Organization trainings instruct attendees on how to create youth-friendly spaces that foster youth empowerment. School trainings instruct attendees on how to improve school climate and create a more solid support system for youth. Youth trainings include bully prevention programs. Community-based trainings include workshops about building community resiliency.

San Jose State University Trainings (408) 924-1000
1 Washington Square, San Jose, CA 95192. www.sjsu.edu. Provides free QPR, ASIST and A Thousand Stars trainings. For information on in-person and online QPR training, contact Dr. Lee at Wei-Chien.Lee@sjsu.edu.

BAY AREA

Bay Area Suicide and Crisis Intervention Alliance (BASCIA)
www.bascia.org. Offers online educational resources and events throughout the year.

Greater San Francisco Bay Area Chapter of the
American Foundation for Suicide Prevention (707) 968-7563
2471 Solano Avenue, Suite 114, Napa, CA 94558.www.afsp.org. Offers online webinars and video libraries to educate AFSP's sui-

---

Important Suicide-Related Resource Not Listed?

Please contact me and let me know. Email info@merrittmental-health.com or call 415-285-3774.

Factors That Mitigate Risk

- Removal of means
- Compassionate listening, validation, and support
- Suicide risk treatment planning
- Reduction of acute stressors
- Compliance with medications and psychotherapy
- Treating depression and substance use disorders
- Close relationships and community
- Instilling hope and processing grief
- Meaningfulness and purpose
- Acknowledgement of illness
- Abstinence from psychoactive substances
- Credible agreement to follow a Crisis Plan
- Initiation of psychopharmacology specifically directed at reducing suicide risk
- Initiation of psychotherapy specifically directed at reducing suicide risk
- Ongoing assessment and treatment plan revision

cide prevention advocates and other online education for middle school, high school, and college students; physicians, the media, and the community.

Northern California Psychiatric Society (415) 334-2418

77 Van Ness, Suite 101, #2022, San Francisco, CA 94102. www.ncps.org. Offers educational lectures and other events throughout the year for psychiatrists and other mental health professionals.

NATIONAL

Suicide Awareness Voices of Education (SAVE) (952) 946-7998 www.save.org. Provides school-based programs, professional trainings, and community presentations. Offers a "Let's Talk About It" event anywhere in the nation. This community public awareness event is designed to give families and community members answers to mental health, mental wellness, and suicide prevention questions. Panel discussions are presented by students and adults, with a question and answer period. To host this event in your community, contact Linda Mars, Event Coordinator at lmars@save.org.

13

Suicide Prevention Apps

Online technology is expanding at a breakneck pace never before seen in 5000 years of technological advancement since the invention of iron smelting and hieroglyphics. Is it a bubble? Are we rushing headlong towards this new, new thing blindly and impulsively, like lemmings headed for the cliff?

Especially in the field of suicide prevention, we must be cautious. Machines can do much, but they cannot replace human beings in the art of empathic listening and the development of the trust and hope that lie at the heart of suicide prevention.

Can machines care? They can, we know, vocalize the language of empathy, but can they be empathic in a manner that touches, transforms, and restores? There are, no doubt, technologists and robotics researchers in Silicon Valley who enjoy to debate these provocative questions. However, let us for the moment dismiss the debate out of hand in reference to suicide prevention.

In this sensitive art and science, the place of machines is: 1) to teach us systematic steps in risk assessment and management and 2) to connect patients, family members, clinicians, educators, and others concerned about suicide risk with helpful, knowledgeable human beings. Machines are the bridge—not the solution.

In this chapter you will find more than a dozen suicide-related apps that are bridges to learning and connection with others. There are general apps for all ages; demographic-specific apps for youths, the elderly, veterans, and the LGBTQ community; screening apps; training apps; crisis line apps; tracking apps; connector apps; and others.

Read the descriptions beneath each entry to determine which app is right for you. Download one.

If you are not certain which to choose—and your aim is to learn how to *Talk About It* warmly and effectively—start with "Suicide Safe" by SAMHSA. Download it. Click on "Conversation Starters." Spend ten minutes reading the authors' wise advice on this topic and navigate from there to case studies, crisis lines, a treatment locator, and more.

Apps are a great way to keep learning and get connected.

Ask and Prevent Suicide

An app using best practices from the ASK (Ask About Suicide) prevention training program. Provides list of warning signs for gauging suicide risk and steps to take if a friend, co-worker, or family member appears at risk. Offers crisis lines focused on veterans and LGBTQ individuals as well as resources for Spanish speakers.

Depression Screening

An app that helps users measure their depression. Assesses user depression in the nine categories of the PHQ-9 diagnostic scale. Enables user to email results to self or clinician. Offers treatment suggestions.

Depression Check

An interactive app developed by M-3 information, the same company that created "What'sMyM3?" (see below). Begins with a short series of questions asking about user's psychological state. Based on the answers, users are given a psychological assessment and suggestions for finding help, as needed.

Did Someone You Know Suicide?

An app for people who have experienced the suicide of a friend or family member. Helps re-direct user's thoughts through a video dialog with a psychologist. Includes contact information for local crisis services.

Hello Cruel World

An app that seeks to alleviate users' suffering by helping them follow their fancies. Provides 101 activities, such as cooking and exercising, for the user. Helps engage the user with the outside world, offering a broader and healthier perspective to their problems.

Help Prevent Suicide

An app using best practices from the Healthy Education for Life Program (HELP). Provides list of warning signs for suicide risk and suggestions for how to talk to those at risk. Includes prevention resources in both Oklahoma, where HELP is based, and nationally.

Is S/O Suicidal?

An app geared toward crisis intervention. Features a video connection to a psychologist who walks the user through numerous interactions. Stands for "Is Someone Suicidal?"

Lifebuoy: Suicide Prevention: Continuity of Care and Prevention

An app for people who have survived a recent suicide attempt. Tries to pre-empt future suicide attempts by helping users track their moods and become more aware of warning signs. Provides ample and easily-accessible information on local resources, including treatment centers and chat lines. Informs users of local events that will take them out of isolation.

Operation Reach Out

An app for both people with suicidal ideation and those trying to help them. Features videos offering solace and instruction for those at risk of suicide. Provides numbers for suicide hotlines. Focuses on military families, but can be used by anyone.

ReliefLink

An award-winning app developed by Emory University. Enables users to create a detailed mental health profile and track their moods in order to become more self-aware. Includes a map locating the nearest mental health resources as well as nearest music options, mindfulness exercises, and other coping mechanisms.

R U Suicidal?

An app for people with suicidal ideation. Provides video excercizes led by a psychologist to offer comfort to users. Helps users monitor their moods over time.

SafeTALK Wallet Card

An app mirroring the function of the safeTALK card given to people over 15 who have passed safeTALK training courses. Uses GPS to track KeepSafe Connections. KeepSafe Connections provide immediate assistance and direct users with suicidal ideation to helpful resources. Available for iPhone and Android.

SAFE-T Method
Suicide Assessment 5-Step Evaluation & Triage

Message to clinicians: What is most important in the assessment and management of suicide risk is that you develop and hone your own systematic approach. If you are looking for a straightforward yet comprehensive template, one of the most widely validated and practiced is the SAFE-T Method, originally developed by Douglas Jacobs, M.D., in collaboration with the National Suicide Prevention Lifeline. It is presented here in abbreviated form. The method is widely available online. You can order a free laminated pocket guide for clinicians at the SAMHSA Store (http://store.samhsa.gov). The method:

1. IDENTIFY RISK FACTORS

☐ Suicidal behavior: history of prior suicide attempts, aborted suicide attempts, or self-injurious behavior.

☐ Current/past psychiatric disorders: especially mood disorders, psychotic disorders, alcohol/substance abuse, ADHD, TBI, PTSD, Cluster B personality disorders, conduct disorders (antisocial behavior, aggression, impulsivity). Co-morbidity and recent onset of illness increase risk.

☐ Key symptoms: anhedonia, impulsivity, hopelessness, anxiety/panic, insomnia, command hallucinations.

☐ Family history: of suicide, attempts or Axis 1 psychiatric disorders requiring hospitalization.

☐ Precipitants/Stressors/Interpersonal: triggering events leading to humiliation, shame or despair (e.g., loss of relationship, financial or health status—real or anticipated). Ongoing medical illness (esp. CNS disorders, pain). Intoxication. Family turmoil/chaos. History of physical or sexual abuse. Social isolation.

☐ Change in treatment: discharge from psychiatric hospital, provider or treatment change.

☐ Access to firearms.

Continued

2. IDENTIFY PROTECTIVE FACTORS

Protective factors, even if present, may not counteract significant acute risk

☐ Internal: ability to cope with stress, religious beliefs, frustration tolerance.

☐ External: responsibility to children or beloved pets, positive therapeutic relationships, social supports.

3. CONDUCT SUICIDE INQUIRY

Specific questioning about thoughts, plans, behaviors, intent

☐ Ideation: frequency, intensity, duration—in last 48 hours, past month, and worst ever.

☐ Plan: timing, location, lethality, availability, preparatory acts.

☐ Behaviors: past attempts, aborted attempts, rehearsals (tying noose, loading gun) vs. non-suicidal self injurious actions.

☐ Intent: extent to which the patient (1) expects to carry out the plan and (2) believes the plan/act to be lethal vs. self-injurious; Explore ambivalence: reasons to die vs. reasons to live.

☐ For youths: Ask parent/guardian about evidence of suicidal thoughts, plans, or behaviors as well as changes in mood, behaviors or disposition.

4. DETERMINE RISK LEVEL/ INTERVENTION

☐ Assessment of risk level is based on clinical judgment after completing steps 1-3.

☐ Reassess as patient or environmental circumstances change.

5. DOCUMENT

☐ Risk level and rationale; treatment plan to address/reduce current risk (e.g., setting, medication, psychotherapy, E.C.T., contact with signifi cant others, consultation); firearm instructions, if relevant; follow up plan. For youths, treatment plan should include roles for parent/guardian.

Stay Alive

An app developed by Grassroots Suicide Prevention, a UK-based charity. Provides a safety plan, a personalized list of reasons to live, and a "life box" where the user can keep photos of important people in their lives.

Suicide or Survive

An app helping users become more self-aware of their individual psychological processes. Provides a mindfulness diary and helpful videos. Helps users monitor their mental well-being over time. Offers information on wellness workshops.

Suicide Safe by SAMSHA

An app made by SAMSHA (the Substance Abuse and Mental Health Services Administration). Provides suicide prevention tips for clinicians based on nationally-recognized standards. Also includes crisis line numbers and guidelines for speaking to families of those at risk of suicide.

Suicide Safer Home

An app helping users try to suicide-proof their home. Provides information on gun and medication storage as well as other suicide prevention measures. Assists mental health professionals, first responders, and people that have a friend at risk of suicide. Includes a scheduler to remind users of safety-related tasks.

Teen Hotlines

An app providing a wide variety of hotlines for teens, parents, and professionals who work with teens. Offers hotlines for teens dealing

---

Advice to Health Professionals

- When in doubt, reach out and *Talk About It*
- Consult with colleagues, hotlines, mobile crisis
- Check your thinking
- *Talk About It* until you feel confident and calm

with eating disorders, depression, substance abuse, and bullying. Includes information on both state and local resources.

What'sMyM3?

An app helping users assess their mental health status in a three-minute test. Provides a score to help users track the sources of any mental health issues. Users can take the test every week to monitor progress.

You are Important: Depression, Suicide, and Bullying Prevention Videos

An app for LGBTQ teens. Features videos from LGBTQ artists, celebrities, business leaders, and public servants that seek to normalize the users' orientation and reinforce their worth as a human being. Based on the It Gets Better® Project and the You Can Play® Project.

14

Experts

Shame, stigma, and a lack of knowledge and understanding of mental illness. These are deeply-rooted cultural trappings that keep us silent and skittish about suicide risk.

A depressed individual thinking of suicide is often profoundly ashamed and either unaware of the presence of mental illness or addiction *as causative* or uninformed about the power of treatment to restore hope and heal. Therefore, what is needed most to prevent suicide is culture change: destigmatization, public education, and national conversation.

As we *Talk About It*, the truth emerges. Thoughts of suicide are uniquely human. They are a paradoxical aspect of human self-consciousness, self-awareness, and death-awareness. We contemplate our existence. We wonder. We imagine. We seek solutions to problems. We seek release from pain. In persisting anguish, healthy people will ponder suicide as one possible escape route from seemingly intractable pain.

As the conversation continues, however, we begin to examine the anguish itself—this is the root cause of suicidal thinking, not existence itself. Wisely, we turn from philosophy to brain science as we recognize that at a certain threshold states of anguish, depression, helplessness, hopelessness, addiction, mania, paranoia, self-hate, guilt, and shame are *mental illnesses*.

Through science, compassion, and attentiveness to suffering, we recognize that these illnesses deserve the same framework of treatment as cancer, diabetes, heart disease, and physical injury. They are illnesses, not lifestyles or metaphysical approaches to the complexities of existence.

To prevent suicide, we must get the word out. Crucially, as a first step, shame must be overcome. Dialogue must commence. Treatment exists. Treatment works. If one form of treatment does not provide someone with relief and hope, he or she must try another. Treat the anguish, the hopelessness, and the depression—successfully—and the suicide risk will dissipate unawares.

The basic message of a national suicide prevention campaign is straightforward: The anguish is not your fault. Seek help. Turn to others. *Talk About It.*

It bears repeating that a fundamental, irreplaceable component of suicide prevention is listening. To help, listen, and keep listening, compassionately. Respond with soft, kind, and supportive words; then reignite the power of listening.

It is through talking and listening that stigma, shame, and suicide lose their hold and power over us.

One way to promote these essential aims of shame and stigma mitigation is through research, lectures, trainings, and conferences. The Bay Area experts listed in this chapter are making unique contributions in the field of suicide prevention.

It is my hope that this chapter will serve as a springboard for public collaborations that help move us out of shame and stigma into fierce honesty, understanding, and effective treatment.

SAN FRANCISCO

Nazneen Bahrassa, Ph.D. (707) 569-239
nazneen.bahrassa3@va.gov. Psychologist for Suicide Prevention Team of the San Francisco VA Medical Center.

Winston Chung, M.D. (415) 600-5739
2340 Clay Street, 7th Floor, San Francisco, California 94115. www.cpmc.org. Medical Director of the CPMC inpatient unit.

Kevin Hines (415) 377-4093
kevin@kevinhinesstory.com. Survivor of a suicide attempt on the Golden Gate Bridge. Best-selling author of *Cracked Not Broken, The Kevin Hines Story*. Public speaker advocating for mental health around the world. Featured in the film *The Bridge*.

Descartes Li, M.D. (415) 476-7448 (415) 285-3774
401 Parnassus Ave, Langley Porter, San Francisco CA 94143. descartes.li@ucsf.edu. Clinical Professor in the Department of Psychiatry at the University of California, San Francisco (UCSF). His roles include Director, UCSF Bipolar Disorder Program; Director, UCSF Electroconvulsive Therapy Service; Director, Brain, Mind, and Behavior; Site Director, Parnassus Campus, Department of Psychiatry Residency Training Program. Gives talks and presentations on mental health in academic and community settings.

Eli Merritt, M.D. (415) 285-3774
3786 20th Street, San Francisco, CA 94110. info@merrittmentalhealth.com. Founder of Merritt Mental Health and a care navigation practice that helps patients find the best care in our fragmented mental health system. Offers lectures and workshops on suicide prevention strategies.

Eve Meyer, MSW, MHSA (415) 984-1900 Ext. 101
P.O. Box 191350, San Francisco, CA 94119-1350. www.sfsuicide.org. Executive Director of San Francisco Suicide Prevention. Frequent spokesperson on suicide prevention and intervention.

Factors & Signs Protective Against Suicide

- Clearly expressed reasons for living
- Resilient or optimistic view of self and future
- Strong family and community connections and supports
- Feelings of responsibility toward others
- Empathetic objections to suicide as harmful to family and friends
- Work/academic/housing stability
- Cultural and religious beliefs that discourage suicide
- Skills in problem solving and conflict resolution
- Good health and access to health care

Melissa Nau, M.D.

1001 Potrero Avenue, SFGH 5, San Francisco, CA 94143. melissa.nau@ucsf.edu. Director of Psychiatric Emergency Services at SF General Hospital. Assistant Professor of Psychiatry at UCSF School of Medicine.

Esme Shaller, Ph.D. (415) 476-7500

401 Parnassus Avenue, San Francisco, CA 94143. Psychologist at UCSF's Langley Porter Psychiatric Institute's Young Adult and Family Center (YAFC). Specializes in treating acute and multi-stressed adolescents in inpatient, residential care, and alternative high school settings. Expert in cognitive and behavioral therapy.

Gifford Boyce-Smith, M.D. (415) 752-2489

50 Beale Street, San Francisco, CA 94105. Board President of NAMI San Francisco.

NORTH BAY

Ryan Ayers (707)968-7563

2471 Solano Avenue, Suite 114, Napa, CA 94558. sfbayarea@afsp.org. Director of the Northern California Chapter of the American Foundation for Suicide Prevention.

Suicide Expert Missing?

Please contact me and let me know. Email info@merrittmental-health.com or call (415) 285-3774.

PENINSULA

Bruce Bongar, Ph.D. (650) 433-3837

bongar@paloaltou.edu Suicidologist. Calvin Professor of Psychology at Palo Alto University. His research and published work focuses on suicide and life-threatening behaviors.

Shashank V. Joshi, M.D. (650) 723-5511

401 Quarry Road, MC 5719, Stanford, CA 94305. svjoshi@stanford.edu. Professor of Child and Adolescent Psychiatry at Stanford.

BAY AREA

Kevin Briggs 1-800-991-6714

KevinBriggs@pivotal-points.com. Former California Highway Patrol Officer. As an officer he dissuaded two hundred people from jumping from the Golden Gate Bridge. Gives public talks about suicide prevention. Promotes mental illness awareness and works to reduce stigma.

15

Bereavement Resources

This book's primary areas of focus are suicide risk assessment and management, resources, and the inordinate value of *Talk About It* as a primary pathway towards the reduction of shame and stigma and the corresponding increase in awareness, education, and prevention.

When suicide does happen, it is a tragedy on at least two levels. One is the premature, sudden loss of a brother, sister, mother, father, friend, or child. The other is the special circumstance of death by suicide, with its unique attendant features of shame, guilt, blame, existential perplexity, and, at times, reenactment by successive generations. Almost always, the grief of suicide is a "complex grief."

This list of bereavement resources is by no means exhaustive. It is meant primarily to remind family and friends who lose someone to suicide that abundant resources do exist to reduce shame and self-blame and, more generally, to aid the grieving process over time.

After suicide, the counsel remains the same: *Talk About It.*

SAN FRANCISCO

San Francisco Suicide Prevention (415) 288-7118

P.O. Box 191350, San Francisco, CA 94119. www.sfsuicide.org. Offers eight-week, peer-led grief support groups for suicide survivors. Graduates of the grief groups can continue to attend support groups on a drop-in basis. Those who have worked through their grief can join Survivors in Action Against Suicide (SAAS), a volunteer program that fights suicide.

Honoring Our Perseverance
and Empowerment (HOPE) (415) 421-2926, ext. 306

870 Market Street, Suite 781, San Francisco, CA 94102. www.namisf.org. Free support group for people who have survived a suicide attempt organized by people who have attempted suicide. Peer-run, weekly group is 12 weeks in duration and includes training in the Wellness Action Recovery Plan (WRAP).

The Compassionate Friends (415) 285-0430

2345 24th Avenue San Francisco, CA 94116 http://www.afsp.org. Free monthly self-help meetings held year-round on the second Wednesday of each month. Open group that can be joined any time. Focus on parents and adult siblings of suicide victims. Local chapter of a national group with no religious affiliation facilitated by a fellow loss survivor.

Center for Elderly Suicide Prevention and
Grief Related Service (415) 750-4180, Ext. 230

3330 Geary Blvd, 3 East, San Francisco, CA 94118. Provides eight-week support group on Wednesday evenings and the last Friday of each month. Graduates are allowed to stop in at future classes on an ongoing basis. Also offers a drop-in, traumatic loss group which occurs Saturday mornings from 10:30 a.m. to 12:30 p.m.

Elements of Management

- Safety
- Appropriate level of care
- Removal of access to means
- Crisis stabilization
- A treatment plan
- Psychotherapy & pharmacology
- Suicide risk tracking

EAST BAY

Survivors of Suicide/Oakland 1-800-260-0094

P.O. Box 3120, Oakland, CA 94609. Support group with regularly-scheduled meetings facilitated by a suicide loss survivor. Group is open; people can join at any time. Sponsored by the Crisis Support Services of Alameda County.

Survivors of Suicide Loss/Oakland (510) 502-6492

Free support group that meets regularly, year-round. Open format allows people to join at any time.

Survivors after Suicide/Walnut Creek (925) 939-1916

P.O. Box 3364 Walnut Creek, CA 94598 www.crisis-center.org. Support group for people who have lost a friend or loved one to suicide. Sponsored by the Contra Costa Crisis Center.

Suicide Attempter Survivor's Guide (510) 420-2475

North Oakland. www.crisissupport.org. Free weekly support group for people who have survived suicide attempts. Open to people 18 and over who are currently in therapy. Sponsored by the Crisis Support Center.

Advice to Health Professionals

- Your own evidence-informed, systematic approach to risk assessment and management is the best approach
- Have a written procedural roadmap at your fingertips ready to review and use at short notice

NORTH BAY

Survivors of Suicide Loss (707) 535-5780

110 Stony Point Road, Suite 110, Santa Rosa, CA 95401. Support group for survivors of suicide victims led by MFTs through Sutter, VNA & Hospice. Meetings held on Mondays between 12:00 p.m. to 1:30 p.m. Also sponsors Kids Together for children ages 5-12 and Teenagers Living with Loss for youth ages 13-17.

Hospice of Petaluma
and Memorial Hospice (707) 778-6242, ext. 322

416 Payran Street, Petaluma, CA 94952. Free support group serving Sonoma and Marin county residents. Facilitated by professionals with personal experience in suicide.

Survivors of Suicide/Novato (415) 260-9864

7 Hayford Court, Novato, CA 94949. Support group for parents whose children have committed suicide. Open format which allows people to join at any time. Meetings from 7:00 p.m. to 9:00 p.m. on the first Tuesday of each month.

PENINSULA

Survivors of Suicide Palo Alto (650) 321-5272

457 Kingsley Avenue, Palo Alto, CA 94301. Free peer-facilitated support group serving San Mateo and Santa Clara counties. Call for times and locations.

Essential Goal of Treatment

The ultimate goal must be to engage the patient in a therapeutic relatiionship.

The Aeschi Working Group

SOUTH BAY

Survivors of Suicide San Jose (408) 885-6216

828 South Bascom Avenue, San Jose, CA 95128. Free support group that meets in eight-week sessions, two hours at a time, on Mondays between 6:30 p.m. and 8:00 p.m. Affiliated with Santa Clara Suicide & Crisis Service.

Survivors of Suicide at The Bill Wilson Center (408) 243-0222

3490 The Alameda, Santa Clara, CA 95050. www.billwilsoncenter.org. Support group for people who have lost a friend or family member to suicide. Held on Saturdays between 12 p.m. - 1:30 p.m.

16

Other Resources

This chapter represents the bright hope of the Suicide Risk Project started in 2014—that is, growth and expansion to include more and more resources dedicated to the mission of increasing awareness, treating suicide risk, and preventing death. Our intent is to publish a second edition of *Suicide Risk in the Bay Area* in 2017.

Let this chapter be an open invitation to any reader to contact us to suggest new ways to achieve these goals and new resources to share with professionals, families, and friends in future editions of the book. As resources accumulate, new directions will become clear. New chapters will form. New collaborations will take shape.

Contact us through the Merritt Mental Health website or email info@merrittmentalhealth.com to share your thoughts, make recommendations, and *Talk About It* any time.

EAST BAY

Bay Area Icarus Project Icarus-oakland@lists.riseup.net

2278 Telegraph Avenue, Oakland, CA 94612. www.theicarusproject.net. A local chapter of the national organization. Provides peer support groups for people with serious mental health challenges by empowering people to name the conditions and process for their recovery on their own terms.

East Bay Agency for Children PALS Program (510) 531-7551

303 Van Buren Avenue, Oakland, CA 94610. www.ebac.org. An in-school counseling program offered to low-income students. Provides 1-on-1 counseling, suicide assessments, and interventions when necessary.

PEERS Oakland (510) 832-7337

333 Hegenberger Road. Oakland, CA 94621. Monday to Friday: 8:30 a.m. to 5:00 p.m. www.peersnet.org. A peer-led organization endeavoring to reduce mental illness stigma and create a space for recovery and wellness. Provides a community support and healing. Offers WRAP groups.

NORTH BAY

People Empowering People (PEP) (707) 259-8692

3281 Solano Avenue, Napa, CA 94558. www.pep-cof.org. A peer-led organization providing group therapy, employment readiness, recovery support, and more. Offers WRAP groups.

Parting Thought

If there is any one secret of success it lies in the ability to get the other person's point of view and to see things from their angle as well as your own.

Henry Ford

PENINSULA

Voices of Recovery (650) 802-6552

310 Harbor Boulevard, Belmont, CA 94002 www.voicesofrecovery-sm.org. A peer-based organization for people needing support guiding their recovery from addiction or from a loved one's addiction. Offers WRAP groups.

BAY AREA

Northern California Psychiatric Society
Wellness Committee (415) 334-2418

77 Van Ness Avenue, Suite 101, #2022, San Francisco, CA 94102. www.ncps.org. Provides consultation and referrals to physicians at risk of suicide. Concerned family members are welcome to call.